ADULT EDUCATION AND HEALTH

Edited by Leona M. English

What are the connections between health and adult learning? What does it mean to move from knowledge about clinical practice in areas such as dietetics, occupational health, nutrition, nursing, medicine, and respiratory technology to the community, higher education settings, and continuing education programs for health professionals?

This collection brings together an interdisciplinary group of scholars and practitioners from health and adult education to address how teaching and learning practices such as participatory planning, storytelling, teamwork, and community mobilization can be used to increase health in the community. The twenty-nine contributors from several continents examine the connections between health and learning and bring both theoretical and practical knowledge to bear on their chapters. This volume provides the missing link to an integrated adult health learning framework, and will serve as a useful introduction to areas such as interprofessional learning, community health education, health policy, First Nations and health, and teaching health professionals.

LEONA M. ENGLISH is a professor in the Department of Adult Education at St Francis Xavier University.

Adult Education and Health

EDITED BY LEONA M. ENGLISH

UNIVERSITY OF TORONTO PRESS
Toronto Buffalo London

© University of Toronto Press 2012
Toronto Buffalo London
www.utppublishing.com
Printed in Canada

ISBN 978-1-4426-4024-5 (cloth)
ISBN 978-1-4426-0998-3 (paper)

Printed on acid-free, 100% post-consumer recycled paper with
vegetable-based inks.

Library and Archives Canada Cataloguing in Publication

Adult education and health / edited by Leona M. English.

Includes bibliographical references.
ISBN 978-1-4426-4024-5 (bound).   ISBN 978-1-4426-0998-3 (pbk.)

1. Public health – Study and teaching (Continuing education).
2. Health education.   3. Adult education.   I. English, Leona

RA440.A38 2012   613'.0715   C2012-900023-X

 Canada Council   Conseil des Arts
for the Arts   du Canada

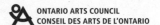 ONTARIO ARTS COUNCIL
CONSEIL DES ARTS DE L'ONTARIO

University of Toronto Press acknowledges the financial assistance to its
publishing program of the Canada Council for the Arts and the Ontario Arts
Council.

University of Toronto Press acknowledges the financial support of the
Government of Canada through the Canada Book Fund for its publishing
activities.

In loving memory of my brother Gerard W. English, 1965–2006

Contents

Part IV: Conclusion

Acknowledgments

The idea for this book began to germinate in the mid-1990s when I came to teach in the Master of Adult Education program at St Francis Xavier University. So many of my graduate students, then and now, were either health professionals or adult educators interested in issues concerning health. I want to thank them for stimulating my own thoughts on the links between health and learning, and for their constant questioning of adult education concepts and ideas. I would also like to acknowledge the strong health and learning community that has emerged around this university, a critical mass of researchers and community developers who want to link health and factors affecting health such as gender, poverty, and literacy. Through their unending dedication to community matters, they have stimulated great interest in this area and given me a creative and invigorating context in which to work.

ADULT EDUCATION AND HEALTH

Introduction

This book arises at a time when many health professionals are developing an interest in adult learning and its connections to the community, as well as its connections to continuing and professional education. They are increasingly aware that education and learning are key in the struggle to promote health in the general population. Indeed, the population at large is realizing that responsibility and ownership of health resides in the community, and that health is affected not only by biology but also by a diversity of social and cultural factors such as education, gender, geography, and employment. Yet, the links between health and education are not always clear either to health professionals or to adult educators engaged in health related practice.

This book-length treatment of health and adult education addresses key questions such as: What are the links between health and adult learning? What does it mean to move from knowledge about clinical practice in areas such as dietetics, occupational health, nutrition, nursing, medicine, and respiratory technology, to the community, higher education settings, and continuing education programs for health professionals? Although health professionals have considerable information on health there is less available to them on health and learning, and more specifically on how to increase the links between health and learning. This gap in knowledge and practice is also apparent to adult educators working with graduate students from the health profession as they delve into adult education theory and practice, and want to use these insights to inform their health practice. For many, the participatory and engaged aspects of adult education are a good fit with their preferred ways of practice. As a consequence, they are interested in learning more about the theory and practice of educating other professionals and the public about health. This book provides the missing link to an integrated adult health learning framework that has a strong theoretical basis.

This collection brings together an interdisciplinary group of scholars and practitioners from health and adult education to answer the question of how teaching and learning practices such as participatory planning, storytelling, teamwork, and community mobilization can be used to increase health in the community and in higher education. The contributors, distinguished in their ability to combine the insights of both health and adult education in their writing and practice, clearly enunciate the links, raise questions, and give examples of their practice. For all their commonality, however, there is a diversity of views represented here: some authors are located only in higher education and others are deeply rooted in the community; others work in clearly identifiable adult education situations such as mentoring junior professionals; while others practice informal strategies such as storytelling and citizen mobilization. This range allows for new and innovative ways of increasing health through an adult learning perspective.

The breadth of perspectives in this text is represented in the authors' diverse understandings of adult education as a field of study and practice. Whereas adult education embraces formal teaching and learning in higher-education classrooms, it also includes informal teaching and learning in the community, such as when community members and health professionals work together to create new knowledge about environmental factors that influence health, or when workshop sessions are used to treat women in addiction recovery. Everyday teaching and learning through informal means is as much a part of adult education as professional training is. Indeed it is this informal sphere that adult education is most concerned with since it has the potential to reach the grassroots, the people most affected by negative health outcomes. As a result, the range of adult education content and methods represented in this book is wide: it includes health policy formation, social change activism, literacy campaigns, and community participation.

A special feature of this text is that the 29 authors from Australia, Botswana, Canada, and the United States give vivid examples from their own practice to illustrate how they have integrated insights from adult learning into their professional practice. The authors have made a special effort to make this book useful to other instructors and teachers whether in a clinical, higher education, or community setting. In making deliberate links between their professions and adult learning, they have challenged readers to do the same. The authors' first audience is graduate students in areas such community nursing, public health, and adult education who want to understand the links between health and education; the second group includes those health and education professionals who want to improve their teaching and learning practice in community and in higher education, such as allied health professionals, aboriginal community workers, physical therapists, and nursing educators. This book provides an extensive and comprehensive reference for health education as a field of study and practice.

Part I: Contextualizing Health and Adult Education

UNESCO (1997) has observed that adult education has much to offer in providing 'relevant, equitable, and sustainable access to health knowledge' (p. 5). What UNESCO does not say is *how* that might happen in practice, what role the various health professionals might play in that practice, and how that knowledge might ultimately influence and potentially transform the entire population. Since an educated population is a healthier population, it is important to know how that population becomes well educated about health. Part I of this book sets the groundwork for the rest of the book by introducing key educational and health concepts related to educating the population and by making explicit the adult learning approach of this book. Chapter 1 presents a critical theory of adult health learning that advocates strong participatory and community-based approaches to learning about and promoting health.

Part II: Adult Education and Health Professionals in the Community

The primary providers of information about health and education are health professionals, although adult educators may become health educators, as is frequently the case in AIDS/HIV situations, which is noted in several chapters in this text. These health educators operate in settings as various as grassroots movements for HIV prevention in Africa, to public and community health clinics in Canada, to literacy-based initiatives in varied local settings. It is within similar community contexts that the adult education field has accumulated a great deal of experience which it can now offer to health professionals seeking new ways to invigorate and transform their practice. Through informal and incidental teaching and learning practices, adult educators have found ways to work with the community in projects affecting the community's health. In Part II (chapters 2–8) the various authors provide concrete examples of how health can be related to learning in professional contexts in community practice. These authors have a very broad understanding of adult education as reaching beyond the formal walls of classrooms. They are concerned with education that occurs when local insight is honoured and used to co-create new knowledge about health, whether through policy, community development, or informal teaching and learning processes.

In chapter 2 community health educator and researcher Maureen Coady, along with nurse educator and development specialist Colleen Cameron, highlights the use of a community health impact assessment tool called PATH (People Assessing Their Health) to engage local residents in assessing factors that affect their health. They use PATH as an example of how to foster adult and community learning, thereby increasing the community's capacity to control and improve local conditions for a healthier community. In chapter 3 adult health educator Linda Ziegahn looks at the use of community-research partnerships which can help build relationships with community members in order to actively involve them in research that affects their health. Ziegahn compares theories of community-engaged research from the field of health with relevant adult learning theories, and provides illustrations of the need and potential for learning in the formation of academic-community health research partnerships. She proposes a number of areas of learning for those researchers, health professionals, and community members participating in community-engaged research aimed at improving health. This is followed in chapter 4 by community-focused health educator and researcher John P. Egan, who explores the Canadian health context as an exemplar of the move to a stronger community basis for health and learning. He focuses on community as a catalyst in changing health care, and emphasizes the role of adult community education – teaching, learning, co-researching, and activism – since adult education principles have often been an integral part of changing policies and practices, and the strengthening of the health of communities.

Peggy Gabo Ntseane and Bagele Chilisa continue the focus on community in chapter 5 by highlighting the use of indigenous knowledge to strengthen adult health learning. The Botswana-based health researchers and educators argue that the Western approach to health education has failed to influence the health care practices and health behaviour of African people. They hold that this failure can only be addressed successfully if the indigenous knowledge (IK) of Africans is taken into account, because the ethics of care for the sick is context-specific. In chapter 6 Marlene Atleo, who specializes in First Nations research and education, also stresses indigenous knowledge, this time in a Canadian context. She speaks to the health and learning approaches used in First Nations communities and provides examples of how the current health status of many of the people in these communities can be redressed through community partnerships and by working *with* First Nations. In chapter 7 literacy and health specialists Barbara Ronson and Irving Rootman examine the relationship between literacy and health, and the intermediary construct 'health literacy,' which is a primary concern for community-based educators. They observe that the study of these relationships can lead to better practice by adult educators and others working in health related fields.

In chapter 8 Donna Chovanec and Brettany Johnson direct attention to health professionals and community service providers working with women in substance abuse programs. From their extensive backgrounds in social work, adult education, and health research, they review the social context within which women's experiences of substance use are situated and make linkages between education/learning and women's substance use, with a special analysis of the learning dimension in recommended treatment approaches. Collectively the seven chapters in this community section set the basis for a collaborative and adult-centred learning that is further developed in Part III for higher education.

Part III: Educating Health Care Professionals

The third part of this book focuses on those health care professionals who provide both professional and continuing professional education to other health care practitioners, often in higher-education environments. The contexts in each case are different and yet each chapter speaks to how health and education are linked in teaching practice. Notably, each author works to make suggestions for how to strengthen professional education.

Part III opens with distinguished adult educator Stephen Brookfield addressing the theme of educating health professionals in higher education. In chapter 9 he provides insights from the general literature on teaching and learning that can be adapted for the field of health education, and pays particular attention to the characteristics of educators that learners find helpful, and the rhythms of learning that adults exhibit. Brookfield's chapter has great relevance for the ways physiotherapists, laboratory technicians, personal care support workers, and other health professionals educate their patients and clients. In chapter 10 Jane Moseley presents her framework for teaching community-based nursing in a higher-education setting. In this chapter she brings her considerable experience of community-based nursing in rural and northern Canada to help student nurses understand and apply adult education principles when working in the community. Speaking to practitioners in gerontology, in chapter 11 Bill Randall builds on his extensive writing on gerontology and narrative to develop his concept of autobiographical learning, a type of learning that life's numerous transitions invite us to experience, including those of getting ill and growing old. While seldom factored into conceptions of 'healthy aging,' Randall shows that autobiographical learning involves learning about ourselves and from ourselves by examining the stories by which we have understood 'our selves' across the years. Learning to facilitate such learning is central to a mode of person-centred care called *narrative care,* a vital (if unexplored) component of the healing process, whatever our area of practice; for example, nursing, social work, chaplaincy. In chapter 12 Daniel Pratt, Leslie Sadownik, and Sandra Jarvis Selinger, a team composed of teachers and physicians, focus on teaching clinicians in medical settings. They propose five sets of Pedagogical BIASes as lenses through which clinicians can reflect upon their approaches to clinical teaching and help make their teaching practice stronger. In chapter 13 Elizabeth Anne Kinsella, Marie-Ève Caty, Stella Ng, and Karen Jenkins continue the theme of teaching in the health professions with their focus on the use of reflective practice in allied health. Building on their varied experiences as professionals in occupational therapy, speech language pathology, audiology, and nursing the authors highlight ways of becoming a reflective practitioner, as well as some of the potential benefits, challenges, and enablers to reflective practice. In all, these five chapters provide considerable insight into the education of health professionals.

The next three chapters in Part III address various forms of interprofessional learning. In chapter 14 Australian-based physical therapists and health educators Joy Higgs, Franziska Trede, and Megan Smith focus on the education of physical therapists and others in a form of interprofessional education. As they note, education occurs both during therapy and as one mode of practice; for instance, during health promotion. According to these authors, to educate others well requires physical therapists to know about how both they and others learn. In chapter 15 Canadians Brian Gastaldi and Kathryn Hibbert consider a number of competencies that might be incorporated into a program for interprofessional education for sports' health care professionals who will work together in the collective care of their patients. They build on their respective competencies in sports therapy and health and education to make their case. Then in chapter 16 Kathryn Hibbert, Mark Hunter, and William Hibbert use informed biography of three professionals, including a police officer, nurse, and paramedic, to illustrate collaborative interprofessional learning opportunities for pre-service and in-service professionals. The biographies serve as an impetus for learning and reveal a common set of core competencies across the professional disciplines.

Part IV: Conclusion

The concluding chapter draws together the cases that have been presented and discusses the implications for teaching and learning among professional and continuing professional educators.

PART I

Contextualizing Health and Adult Education

1 A Critical Theory of Adult Health Learning

LEONA M. ENGLISH

Adult health learning begins with the notion that everything is health and health is everything. This approach is situated in the theory of social determinants of health (SDOH) (Laverack, 2007), that our health is affected by factors such as the environment, race, food security, gender, work, geography, education, and relationships. SDOH acknowledges that in addition to biology, we are as healthy as our environment and that any effort to address health has to take this larger socio-economic environment into account. SDOH and health promotion theories and strategies encourage the community to continue to be involved in a collective process of large- scale change that will positively affect health (Ledwith, 2001). Adult health learning brings a teaching and learning perspective to this theory and stresses the need to focus on adults as participants, critical thinkers, and agents of change.

As effective as theories such as SDOH are at pointing to the contributing factors affecting health they often do not fully integrate a systematic adult learning component or address the specific ways that change can come about. The theory of health and adult learning that is addressed in this chapter, and carried through many of the chapters in this book, includes a role for adult educators as facilitators of change in how everyday citizens and health professionals think about learning for health. To build this theory, this chapter analyses current knowledge in health, critical theory, and adult learning, and uses this knowledge to build a new theory and practice of critical adult health learning. This theory is premised on the need to recognize the pivotal role that 'critical analysis and action' on the many environmental influences that determine health is also needed (Labonte, 2005, p. 2). In presenting principles and critical areas for inquiry and practice – gender, power, ideology, hegemony – this theory establishes a grounding from which to create curriculum, develop teaching practices, and establish interprofessional networks. This theory informs the strategies and practices articulated in many chapters in this book.

Canada's encounters with the H1N1 (Human swine flu) crisis in 2009 and the Severe Acute Respiratory Syndrome (SARS) in 2002–2003 caused citizens to sit up and take notice; for many of them it was an opportunity to think about their health and vulnerability, as well as their responsibility for their community's well-being. These epidemics were the source of untold but necessary educational campaigns about spreading disease, harm reduction, and cultivating risk. Observers pointed to the need to bring awareness about health into the everyday world, not just in times of crises, and citizens became more concerned about being involved and proactive, yet it was not always clear to them how this might happen. A comprehensive view of health and learning that was both respectful of adults and responsive to their learning needs, as well as forward focused, was needed at this time to prepare for and manage health. Although health information was being given to the public through standard media outlets and through new social media sites and blogs, there was an ongoing need to raise the level of public participation and awareness of health and to continue to move it beyond consumption of facts and information. To some degree this happened, yet there was much to be done. Adult education practice and theory had, and continues to have, much to offer in this struggle to increase participation, learner involvement, and community development for better health.

Arguably, what would be useful is a more complex model of health and learning that integrates a systematic review of theoretical dimensions of health that contribute to learning and vice versa, and uses this review to build a new theoretical and critical framework for adult health learning. Existing models of health education (e.g., Buchanan, 2006) are fine insofar as they have the potential to help adults change or modify lifestyle behaviours (e.g., stop smoking, eat local, avoid overeating, limit salt intake), yet they often do not move to active participation and engagement. This chapter responds to existing models by providing a brief review of the literature on health, as well as on critical theory perspectives such as social class, ideology, power, and race. The result is a theory to fill a knowledge gap around adult learning and health, and to complement existing practices of raising awareness of health issues and promoting individual behaviour change. Given the great number of health professionals writing about learning, this theoretical framework will help to further conceptualize the political and issue-ridden dimensions of learning for health, and help inform critical practices of education for health. This framework is distinguished by its stress on bringing the insights of critical theory to bear on health knowledge and adult education. These three components are discussed in turn and integrated throughout this chapter.

Health Theory

The first body of literature to contribute to a critical theory of adult health learning is health. In particular, the literature on health promotion is used because it has drawn attention to the many ways that health in a community is determined by factors that include both the individual and the larger community (Raphael & Bryant, 2002). These factors include societal structures that influence an individual's sense of control and well being. Health promotion, by and large, is a multidisciplinary response to the narrow health education perspective that dominated up until the 1980s. Health promotion theorists continue to work to inform the public about these social determinants of health since it has become increasingly evident that they affect the health of individuals and communities (Raphael, 2008b, p. 2). Health promotion makes it clear that in order to address health, the public needs to be engaged in a participatory and comprehensive process of identifying and working with social determinants to create change. This approach coincides with the reformer perspective outlined by Pratt, Sadownik, and Jarvis Selinger later in this text. Given adult education's strength in community development, adult learning and activism would seem to be ready contributors to health promotion, and have the potential to make major changes.

One of the key determinants of health within the social determinants of health framework is education (Raphael, 2008b). Studies of participation show that people with higher levels of education and health are more likely to participate further in formal higher education, and they are more likely to engage in lifelong learning pursuits (Feinstein & Hammond, 2004). Well educated citizens are also more likely to volunteer and to participate in the life and governance of their communities (Mundel & Schugurensky, 2008). Beyond the benefits of education, it is generally recognized that the mere fact of engaging in lifelong learning contributes to health. According to a report from the Center for Research on the Wider Benefits of Learning, 'Participation in adult learning contributes to positive and substantial changes in health behaviors and small improvements in wellbeing' (Feinstein, Hammond,

Woods, Preston, & Bynner, 2003, p. iv; Feinstein & Hammond). This is good news for adult educators who have known this fact intuitively for sometime but now have it verified.

Yet, despite the insights of health promotion theory, some of the health and learning literature is limited to treating illness and curing patients (Hill & Ziegahn, 2010). The arena envisaged in a critical theory of adult learning is larger – it embraces the whole community in assessing and promoting their health. Consequently, a health promotion approach moves the focus from reliance on health education literature when one is sick, to community engagement in health promotion activities such as community kitchens, faith-based health programs, and environmental campaigns, as an everyday occurrence.

Yet, while the health promotion literature suggests change, it sometimes does not go far enough in embracing an adult learning model. The type of health and learning approach that is envisaged here is well illustrated in a small university town in Nova Scotia. An intercommunity and interagency partnership has emerged in which health promotion advocates have come together with librarians, developers, sustainability advocates, and citizenship groups to build a centralized learning centre called the People's Place, which includes a town library; space for literacy programs, non-profit group meetings and youth gatherings; as well as a health education resource centre, community kitchen, and community food security space. This is an integrative approach that sees health as an important aspect of life in the community and as one that is intricately tied to health and learning. And it is here that health promotion advocates and community developers find common vision and create new alternatives for healthy communities.

Significantly, many of the insights about health promotion were well established even before documents such as the Ottawa Charter (World Health Organization, 1986) made health promotion a well known concept. Many in the health professions know at least at an intuitive level that adult learning is linked to their practice. Those who enter graduate adult education programs, like authors Moseley and Sadownik (this volume), often want to look at their professional practice in new ways. Some, such as dieticians and pharmacists, are aware of the socio-cultural dimensions of health and know that their work in community is about educating for change. Often they work in public health roles and teach informally on a daily basis. The question for them and for many in adult education is: How are health and learning related, and how do I move to a bottom-up and more comprehensive view of health?

Critical Theory

The critical social sciences help to probe the philosophy of practice that engages the determinants of health and which helps learners move beyond the basic teaching and learning processes. The Marxian-informed perspective of critical theory allows us to work with a broad-based social and political approach (Allman, 2000) to contribute to a theory of adult health learning. A centerpiece of this theory, as Brookfield (2005; this volume) notes, is its learning tasks, which show that not only is the content of learning reformed but so are the structures that undergird it. Brookfield names the learning challenges of critical theory as 'learning to challenge ideology, contest hegemony, unmask power, overcome alienation, learn liberation, reclaim reason, and practice democracy' (2005, p. 2). These learning tasks are integrated into this proposed theory of health and learning, along with understandings of gender and race. These are intended to foster the development of insights to address inequalities. For the engaged adult educator, these are all teaching tasks for increased community health. Below, the salient aspects of critical theory are used to illustrate the links to health.

Challenging Ideology

Ideologies (Brookfield, 2005) such as individual-focused health education, professionals as all-knowing purveyors of health, and citizens as consumers of expert medicine have come to dominate the Western world. These ideologies have become hegemonized so that some citizens see themselves subject to the machinery of hospitals and evidence-based medicine in which their health needs are not always met. A revised theoretical approach, rooted in health promotion, works with learners in participatory ways to reclaim health. It also broadens what they learn (e.g., how to quit smoking) to the larger global structures, corporate capitalism, financial regimes, environmental degradation, and corporate downsizing, all of which limit human agency and perspective, and which contribute to the unequal distribution of disease and access to health care (Marmot & Wilkinson, 2006). These ideologies can be addressed through a variety of means starting with citizens becoming better informed about their options and engaged in collective action on the social determinants of health, such as their environment and social location as well as employment status, educational opportunities, and living conditions.

A narrowly defined understanding of health as confined only to professionals and hospitals when one is sick, as important as these are, is an ideology that needs to be addressed. It has led some citizens to focus only on disease and to ignore the social determinants of health which may have contributed to illness. Yet, the signs of hope are growing, especially in terms of awareness of environmental effects on health. Canada is home to a major social movement that protests clear-cutting of our forests and other forms of environmental degradation (Walter, 2007). Social movement learning (Hall & Clover, 2005) within these events is especially poignant in a country which has been built on the resource economies of logging, oil drilling, mining, and fishing. There is growing awareness that the ideologies that seem to undergird most of these resource developments and concomitant effects on our environment are pragmatism, globalization, and capitalism, and that the side effects are sometimes detrimental to healthy living. Public awareness of the SDOH is increasing, as is the recognition of the need to work with learners to identify the ways in which these ideologies have affected the health of our communities. A recent report of the World Health Organization (2008) reinforces that healthy public policy – focused on improving the circumstances in which people are born, grow, live, work, and age.

Challenging Social Class

An ideology rarely succeeds unless it has the support of people and institutions around it. And in this case, regressive models of health have been bolstered by social class issues, which as Mojab (2005) points out, are a major factor in all world events. Social class is the direct result of the situation into which we are born and it affects our identity and how we cope with the world; when class is entwined with issues of race and gender, the situation becomes more complex. In terms of health and learning, class affects who has access to health and education, who controls health and education, and who will benefit most from changes in health and education (see Schecter & Lynch, 2010). Improved social class translates into a higher standard of living, better paying jobs, and access to health care services.

Griff Foley (2005), an adult educator and social movement theorist influenced by Marx, notes that there are preferred and embedded ways of learning for the higher social classes, especially the professional classes: namely, higher education. For the lower social classes learning preferences and choices are limited and are more likely to be located in the community. It is no wonder then that many of our efforts in adult learning are focused on informal and nonformal learning strategies in the community. The historical roots of adult educators are with the grass-roots population and struggling classes, providing them with the expertise to address social class and its effects on health. Of particular concern is that citizens within the lower social and economic strata have more difficulty accessing services including formal education, and consequently may have greater need for adult learning in informal settings. Standard health education models, which are frequently premised on schooling, are insufficient. Knowing where we ourselves are located within the social and economic system, what our privilege consists of, or, to borrow from Peggy McIntosh (2006), to unpack our own knapsack of cultural, social, and economic capital, is necessary for those who work in critical adult health education. Adult education has a long history of negotiating positionality and using it to understand systems and relationships, and to facilitate dialogue on these issues. The issue of food security for instance is a prime starting place for this type of analysis. Who has access to quality food sources and why? How does this affect our long-term health and what are the implications for having a limited supply? Who controls the global food system? Why is a bottle of Coke less expensive than a bottle of orange juice?

Unmasking Power

Classic theories of power are a strong part of critical theory. These theories address the constraints against advancing in the existing system and the struggles that citizens have to resist the holders of power such as departments of health and government officials (Kaufman, 2010). Embedded within these classic notions of power are systems of privilege that limit access to the determinants of health. While health institutions and pharmaceutical corporations can be identified readily, the holders of power outside the health system are more difficult to pinpoint even though they contribute to a complex array of factors that affect health, such as employment, environment, and education. Within education, the holders of power are those who set standards for literacy, grant access, award diplomas, and establish the curriculum for schools and universities, as well as teach. It is not coincidental that these holders of power have typically been educated and socialized through liberal education models.

Traditional health education settings such as public health clinics often have health educators delivering smoking cessation or weight reduction programs; the primary task of these professionals is to transfer knowledge to the community and help change negative behaviours. While this has been an effective strategy it is increasingly complemented by a community-led process, informed by a critical theory of health and learning, proposals in which power is distributed among the group of participants so that the facilitator (who could be a health professional such as a nurse) engages teachers and learners in a participatory process to look not only at disease or negative behaviour but also at issues such as the impact of a box store on a small town with multiple family run businesses. An engaged community health process to address issues of health could examine the effects of unemployment, minimum-wage, and part-time jobs, and loss of markets for locally produced food. In this case, the responsibility is moving to the community and its reservoir of knowledge and ability. The focus is on learning and change. Those with formal educational preparation for the health professions – for example, pharmacists, respiratory technologists, and physicians, many of whom have contributed to this book – might indeed be called on to teach others and contribute their knowledge, but they would be one source among many.

The transition in this renewed system would be from nurse to nurse educator or facilitator, from gerontologist to community developer, from lab technologist to community participant, and so on. Of course, within a medical setting such as a hospital or higher-education classroom these professionals would also fill their official roles, but their arena of practice would become more diffuse and their role would be part of a collective. This broadened model can cause a shift of identity for some health professionals who study adult education or health promotion. While some are disappointed because they want to focus on stronger instructional skills for teaching in higher-education settings such as community college, many embrace the adult education facilitator and program planning roles that encourage participatory and discovery learning.

The diffusion of power within these community settings and within individual roles is often a challenge, but a welcome one for those who are oriented to health promotion and healthy communities. As Foley (2005) has noted, it is the participants' willingness to value and evaluate their own experiences and privilege that helps adult educators most (p. 43). In essence, individuals need to be viewed not as health consumers, as if health services were the source of health, but rather as health creators, recognizing that health is 'won by the people themselves' (Catford, 2004, p. 2). Any effective model of adult learning for health has to take into account this expertise and willingness, especially as it relates to grassroots learning: learning through creativity, the arts, the body, activism, and the everyday world. This is the transformative potential of this critical theory of adult learning.

Gendering and Racializing Learning

An integral part of this critical theory of adult learning is the incorporation of an understanding of the effect of gender and race on adult learning and the health of communities. It is no accident that the people on First Nations reserves in Canada have the lowest health outcomes of all citizens (Reading, 2009). And it is no surprise that they also have the lowest education levels and greatest levels of poverty, which are major determinants of health. Hence the ongoing interest of First Nations in moving beyond traditional health education such as alcohol and tobacco cessation programs and on to health promotion initiatives which address factors affecting their health, namely disease, poverty, education, and environmental degradation. As noted in Atleo's chapter in this book, this shift represents a return to a culturally based view of health which is ecological and holistic.

The experience of women and health is also a focus for this critical theory of adult learning and health. Women's health is a particular issue because women are more likely to suffer ill effects of environmental degradation and economic downturns (Clover, 2003). Moreover, research is increasingly alerting us to the ways that sex and gender interact to create and challenge women's health and well-being (Health Canada, 1999; Hill & Ziegahn, 2010). Chovanec and Johnson probe this theme in their chapter on women and substance abuse. A major question is how to adequately address women's situation in a way that values them as learners and citizens. There are some helpful signs of progress in this area, including the increasing evidence of women coming together to demand better diagnosis and treatment in areas such as breast cancer, and in creating solutions to maternal and child poverty.

Implications for the Education of Adults

Any effective model of critical adult learning for health has to take into account adult education's expertise with grassroots learning, and our knowledge of the integration of creativity, the arts, the body, and activism into the teaching and learning process. All of these factors contribute to an integrative framework that infuses the transformative potential of the theory. Yet, specific strategies and practices for accomplishing some of this transformation are difficult to itemize and explain. This section identifies two key pedagogical strategies as a starting place.

Working in a Participatory Mode

The use of a collective learning model, which many health professionals and adult educators already embrace, is integral to all social learning processes. When groups are facilitated well, the strengths of the whole group can be harnessed for change. One example is the increase in the number of citizens such as the ones described by Coady and Cameron (this volume), who are engaged in a community health impact assessment (CHIA) process in which they meet to assess how changes such as incoming provincial budgets or minimum-wage adjustments will have positive and negative effects on the health of the community. The sceptic might ask what the budget has to do with health; those interested in health promotion know that everything from disposable income, to the food supply, to how the non-profit sector is able to function are connected to health. How the government spends funds affects employment rates, the educational system, and monies for local literacy initiatives. The provincial budget is a matter of health. In a revised adult health learning model there is a need for more groups and more citizen-based models that work with community needs and knowledge.

Working in Higher Education

Adult educators have a role in influencing how education is done in professional health programs. Graduate degree programs provide an opportunity to improve teaching and learning across the disciplines by modelling creative strategies; introducing the concepts of power, hegemony, class, and gender to students; and by encouraging the use of a variety of participatory teaching strategies. Given the amount of content that most professional programs are intended to cover, it is sometimes difficult to include discussion or multiple modes of learning, yet these concepts and practices are important in facilitating change. Although some, such as Bryan, Kreuter, and Brownson (2008), have developed a list of ways (tips) for educating those in health professions, what is being encouraged here is less about teaching tips and more about a philosophy of inclusion, critical thinking, and a broad-based understanding of health which honours interprofessional knowing. When critical perspectives are encouraged then there are challenges to taken-for-granted ideas and practices. In chapter 10 of this volume, Moseley demonstrates how she teaches nursing students in a public health course to work with communities to create solutions. Randall, in chapter 11 on narrative care, looks at how professionals working with the aged might use an autobiographical perspective on care; while Higgs, Trede, and Smith (chapter 14) examine how physical therapists can move from a clinical to an educative role. Indeed, it seems that many creative options are in use and that many are already employing them to increase knowledge of health, to broaden the issues to social and environmental factors, and to encourage critical capacity. While good teachers in any discipline are needed, they are especially needed in areas where the future professional will need to work with the community on matters of health.

These are two strategies and approaches, and obviously they are limited. Yet, they suggest the need to think creatively and broadly about health. Adult educators who have experience in these areas have much to offer in this regard.

Conclusion

There is evidence that this critical theory of health and adult learning is being implemented, though it has not been identified as such. Some very strong voices can be heard, such as Ronson and Rootman (this volume) on the connection between literacy and health, and Denis Raphael (2008a) on the need for a decided stress on health promotion. Yet, it remains for the learning dimension to be further highlighted. The time is ripe for this to happen in order that those concerned about health can continue to create viable community models of living. This chapter has provided a critical and theoretical framework that strengthens their pedagogical and emancipatory practices, and which encourages health for all.

REFERENCES

Allman, P. (2000). *Revolutionary social transformation: Democratic hopes, political possibilities and critical education*. Westport, CT: Bergin & Garvey.

Brookfield, S.D. (2005). *The power of critical theory: Liberating adult learning and teaching*. San Francisco: Jossey-Bass.

Bryan, R.L., Kreuter, M.W., & Brownson, C. (2008). Integrating adult learning principles into training for public health practice. *Health Promotion Practice, 10*, 557–563.

Buchanan, D.R. (2006). A new ethic for health promotion: Reflections on a philosophy of health education for the 21st century. *Health Education and Behaviour, 33*(3), 290–304.

Catford, J. (2004). Health promotion's record card: How principled are we 20 years on? *Health Promotion International, 19*(1), 1–4.

Clover, D.E. (Ed.). (2003). *Global perspectives in environmental adult education.* New York: Peter Lang.

Feinstein, L., & Hammond, C. (2004). The contribution of adult learning to health and social capital. *Oxford Review of Education, 30*(2), 199–221.

Feinstein, L., Hammond, C., Woods, L., Preston, J., & Bynner, J. (2003). *The contribution of adult learning to health and social capital.* Report # 8, London, UK. The Centre for Research on the Wider Benefits of Learning. Available at http://www.learningbenefits.net/Publications/ResReps/ResRep8.pdf.

Foley, G. (2005). Educational institutions: Supporting working-class learning. In T. Nesbit (Ed.), *Class concerns: Adult education and social class* (pp. 37–44). San Francisco: Jossey-Bass.

Hall, B.L., & Clover, D.E. (2005). Social movement learning. In L.M. English (Ed.), *International encyclopedia of adult education* (pp. 584–589). New York: Palgrave Macmillan.

Health Canada. (1999). *Women's health strategy.* Ottawa: Minister of Public Works and Government Services.

Hill, L., & Ziegahn, L. (2010). Adult education for health and wellness. In In C. Kasworm, A. Rose, & J. Ross-Gordon (Eds.), *Handbook of adult and continuing education* (pp. 295–303). Thousand Oaks, CA: Sage.

Kaufman, J.J. (2010). The practice of dialogue in critical pedagogy. *Adult Education Quarterly, 60*(5), 456–476.

Labonte, R. (2005). Editorial: Towards a critical population health research. *Critical Public Health,* 15(1), 1–3

Laverack, G. (2007). *Health promotion practice: Building empowered communities.* New York: Open University Press.

Ledwith, M. (2001). Community work as critical pedagogy: Re-envisaging Freire and Gramsci. *Community Development Journal, 36*(3), 171–182.

Marmot, M., & Wilkinson, R.G. (Eds.). (2006). *Social determinants of health* (2d ed.). New York: Oxford University Press.

McIntosh, P. (2006). White privilege: Unpacking the invisible knapsack. In E. Lee, D. Menkart, & M. Okazawa-Rey (Eds.), *Beyond heroes and holidays* (pp. 83–86). Washington, DC: Network of Educators on the Americas.

Mojab, S. (2005). Class and race. In T. Nesbit (Ed.), *Class concerns: Adult education and social class* (pp. 73–82). San Francisco: Jossey-Bass.

Mundel, K., & Schugurensky, D. (2008). Community based learning and civic engagement: Informal learning among adult volunteers in community organizations. *New Directions for Adult and Continuing Education, 118*: 49-60.

Raphael, D. (2008a). Grasping at straws: A recent history of health promotion in Canada. *Critical Public Health, 18*(4), 483–495.

Raphael, D. (Ed.). (2008b). *Social determinants of health: Canadian perspectives* (2d ed.). Toronto: Canadian Scholars' Press.

Raphael, D., & Bryant, T. (2002). The limitations of population health as a model for a new public health. *Health Promotion International, 17*(2), 189–199.

Reading, J.L. (2009). *The crisis of chronic disease among aboriginal peoples: A challenge for public health, population health and social policy.* Victoria, BC: University of Victoria Centre for Aboriginal Health Research.

Schecter, S.R., & Lynch, J. (2010). Health learning and adult education: In search of a theory of practice. *Adult Education Quarterly,* doi: 10.1177/0741713610380438.

Walter, P. (2007). Adult learning in new social movements: Environmental protest and the struggle for the Clayoquot Sound rainforest. *Adult Education Quarterly, 57*(3), 248–263.World Health Organization. (WHO). (1986). Ottawa charter for health promotion. Retrieved 2 March 2009 from http://www.who.int/hpr/archive/docs/ottawa.html.

World Health Organization (WHO). (2008). Closing the gap in a generation: Health equity through action on the social determinants of health. Retrieved 10 October 2011 from http://whqlibdoc.who.int/hq/2008/WHO_IER_CSDH_08.1_eng.pdf.

PART II

Adult Education and Health Professionals in the Community

2 Community Health Impact Assessment: Fostering Community Learning and Healthy Public Policy at the Local Level

MAUREEN COADY AND COLLEEN CAMERON

Health professionals have come to realize that health policy should be directed at reducing health inequalities (Wilkinson, 1996, 2006), and that education of the public is the key to addressing complex health determinants (Tones & Tilford, 2001). The vision is of individuals and communities who come together to learn from one another, to jointly identify issues of concern to their health and well-being, and to decide on the appropriate plan and actions to address these issues. The practices used in this community process are adult education strategies of organizing, facilitating, and working collectively for change. In line with this vision, this chapter describes Community Health Impact Assessment (CHIA), a learning-based approach that brings the community's voice forward in the discussion of health decision-making and the development of healthy public policy (PATH, 2008). Emerging from the People Assessing their Health (PATH) projects in northeastern Nova Scotia, Canada, CHIA places adult learning at the heart of effective policies and processes. This chapter focuses on this learning dimension, which to date has been given little practical and theoretical consideration (Stuttaford & Coe, 2007), but which is increasingly seen as 'the real catalyst for change' (Simpson & Freeman, 2004, p. 346) in effective health promotion and education programs.

CHIA is an approach that enables citizens to assess the impact of a project, program, or policy on the health of their community. The processes involved provide a concrete way for involved citizens to influence public policy, a theme that is at the heart of Egan's chapter in this book. Our experience is that the engagement of community members in these processes results in informal learning that is transformative. It increases individual and public understanding of the determinants of health, and empowers citizens to play an active role in decisions affecting their health (Mittelmark, 2001). We believe that the collective community knowledge created from this educational interaction strengthens a community's capacity to take action to improve the health and well-being of their community.

This chapter describes the processes and the learning involved, as well as lessons learned from the implementation of a community health impact assessment in different community settings and cultural contexts. The chapter explores CHIA as a highly inclusive and participatory community health development process that can lead to sustainable change at the community level. As an educational process, we argue that CHIA provides an empowerment strategy that can help people make critical value judgments about their priorities and choices and the kind of society in which they want to live (Buchanan, 2006). This chapter will be of interest to health professionals and for graduate students in the health professions, as well as those involved in community health and development.

This chapter will also be of interest to adult and health educators and community development practitioners committed to moving beyond the information-transmission limitations of a health care systems approach, which Pratt, Sadownik, and Selinger also address in chapter 12 in this book. It will also be of interest to policy-makers committed to these ideals and supportive of the involvement of citizens in the development of healthy public policy.

The Healthy Public Policy and Health Impact Assessment Context

Successive global health promotion agreements, most notably the Ottawa Charter for Health Promotion (WHO, 1986) and the Jakarta Declaration on Leading Health Promotion into the 21st Century (WHO, 1997), have advocated building healthy public policy as a key action front for global health development. A *healthy public policy* is a policy that increases the health and well-being of those individuals and communities that it affects (Kemm, 2001). It is oriented to the future state of health, to multiple small-scale solutions, and to the involvement of individuals and the local community in those solutions (Hancock, 1985; Mittelmark, 2001). The emphasis is on refocusing a preoccupation in public policy with the existing sick care system, to a focus on creating health (Hancock & Minkler, 2002). The development of healthy public policy relies heavily on adult learning; it recognizes that people know a great deal about what affects their health, and can be involved in planning action to improve individual and community health. A more recent report of the World Health Organization's Commission on the Social Determinants of Health (WHO, 2008) reinforces that healthy public policy – focused on improving the circumstances in which people are born, grow, live, work, and age – is now more important than ever.

Health impact assessment (HIA) is an essential tool for policy-making and practice. It is a combination of procedures, methods, and tools that systematically judges the effects of a specific action (i.e., policy, program) on the health of a defined population (Barnes & Scott-Samuel, 2000), or a community. It aims to ensure that the health consequences of a policy or decision are considered prior to their implementation (Kemm, 2001), and identifies strategies and action to manage these effects (International Association of Impact Assessment, 2006; Barnes & Scott-Samuel, 2000). Drawing support from environmental impact assessment, the trend to use health impact assessment to support the adoption of healthy public policies has been developing rapidly in the United Kingdom, Southeast Asia, and Australia. In Canada, the most consistent efforts to implement HIA have been in British Columbia between 1993 and 2000, and more recently in Quebec, where, since 2001, all ministries and agencies must make sure their laws and regulations have no significant negative effects on the health and well-being of the population (St-Pierre, 2008). These processes assume learning that informs the development of policies to better meet the needs of the population they are intended to serve.

While governments and non-governmental organizations at various levels generally initiate HIA using their own standardized tools and processes, the People Assessing Their Health (PATH) process, described in this chapter, helps communities initiate and drive their own HIA process, using their own unique community health impact assessment tool (CHIAT). The process that leads to the creation of the tool, called the PATH process, involves learning that enables communities to develop an understanding of health issues and determinants. They learn to think about health in a new way: from the perspective of the community as a whole, rather than just individuals' illnesses. The process of developing and using the tool extends this learning to an understanding of how programs and policies can increase or weaken community health (Mittelmark, 2001). Use of the tool helps communities identify ways to maximize the benefits and minimize the negative effects of a change, policy, or program (PATH, 2007). This learning enables them to become involved in promoting healthy public policy development at a local level.

The History of PATH and the CHIAT

The People Assessing Their Health (PATH) project, or PATH I, emerged in 1996 as a partnership between existing community organizations: a local women's resource centre, a university extension department, a public health services unit, and local community development leaders in northeastern Nova Scotia. PATH was envisioned as a way to stimulate community learning and participation in an emerging regional health system. As PATH developed, however, it became apparent that the dialogue and deliberation processes involved provided diverse opportunities for co-learning between the partnership organizations and the communities involved as they worked together to strategize how the community could have a greater voice in health decision-making and healthy public policy processes. This learning is reported in this chapter.

The project operated in three diverse rural communities in northeastern Nova Scotia. Two part-time project coordinators provided support and training for local facilitators. The facilitators used a variety of adult education and community development techniques to engage people in examining the factors that affect their health and well-being. Each community developed its own community health impact assessment tool, based on the factors that they identified in the PATH process, and tested on hypothetical projects. A regional workshop was held at the conclusion of the work to share outcomes of the projects, and to launch a resource entitled *PATHways to Building Healthy Communities in Northeastern Nova Scotia: The PATH Project Resource* (Gillis, 1997; NCCHPP, 2009).

In 1997, the PATH Network evolved to continue the process of sharing information and providing learning opportunities related to community health and community health impact assessment. The membership comprised the original community partnership organizations, including community-based organizations and universities and community health boards, but also other interested groups and individuals. PATH Network members continue to share a vision of working together to build healthier communities by creating opportunities for all citizens to learn about the broad range of factors that determine their health.

The second PATH project, officially titled Applying Community Health Impact Assessment to Rural Community Health Planning, or PATH II, was initiated by the PATH Network, the Antigonish Women's Resource Centre, and Public Health Services in partnership with the Antigonish Town and Country Community Health Board. The project, launched in 2000, focused on developing and testing a community health impact assessment tool, developed from the community health board's vision of a healthy community. The processes involved helped the community health board members learn more about factors determining health in their community: they also learned how to use a wider range of information for evidence-based decision-making. The resulting CHIAT was tested with three community groups including the local town council, a local breastfeeding group, and the community health board itself. Similar to PATH I (Gillis, 1997), in order to share information and lessons learned in the project, a resource entitled *PATHways II: The Next Steps – A Guide to Community Health Impact Assessment* (PATH, 2002) was produced and widely distributed.

Following the completion of the PATH 1 and PATH II Projects, the PATH Network has been engaged in activities to promote the application of community health impact assessment in a variety of different settings: locally, nationally, and internationally. In 2003 the PATH Process was used by the Association for Social and Health Advancement, based in Kolkata, India, to help a self-help women's group in West Bengal develop their own CHIAT. Again in 2006, the Association for Social and Health Advancement facilitated the PATH process with a tribal community in West Bengal, who were about to embark on an indigenous tourism project initiated by the United Nations Development Program and the Indian government. The following year, this tribal community used their vision of a healthy community to develop their own Peoples' Charter for Sustainable Tourism. Similarly, in the spring of 2009, the Centre for Indigenous Knowledge and Organizational Development in Ghana, Africa, facilitated the PATH process with their staff and associates. They also used their CHIAT to assess the potential impact of an ecological tourism proposal on the health of their communities.

Locally in Nova Scotia, and across Canada, a number of organizations have gone through the PATH process and developed their own CHIAT. In 2008 the Antigonish Town and Country Community Health Board's tool was used by local citizens to assess the potential impact of a large recreation project on the health and well-being of the community; in 2009 a number of community organizations in Saskatoon, Saskatchewan, also learned to conduct the PATH process. Throughout 2009 a third major project of the PATH Network, entitled *Influencing Healthy Public Policy with Community Health Impact Assessment*, has been supported by the National Collaborating Centre for Healthy Public Policy (NCCHPP). The NCCHPP is one of six centres of the Public Health Agency of Canada that was established to provide national focal points for knowledge exchange and dissemination in key areas of public health (St-Pierre, 2008). As part of its efforts to support and promote health impact assessment, the PATH Network was engaged to look at the conditions necessary to support community-driven health impact assessment, and, using that lens, to identify ways to move forward with this work (NCCHPP, 2009).

Concurrent with each of the PATH projects, the PATH Network members have been involved in disseminating knowledge about PATH and community health impact assessment in health, academic, and public policy arenas. Network members have presented papers at national and international conferences, including the World Health Organization's Fifth Global Conference on Health Promotion in Mexico in 2000. More recently, network members have presented papers and participated as resource persons in forums and consultations on health impact assessment in Canada and internationally, including Thailand, Australia, and Ghana.

Adult Learning and the PATH Process

PATH is a simple and highly practical process that provides ordinary people with the knowledge and critical skills to understand the local issues and develop their own plans of action to bring about a change in their present or future health (Cameron, 2009). It incorporates adult education community development strategies, including a focus on the adult learning cycle, the value of experiential learning, and the use of the story dialogue approach (Gillis & English, 2001). These strategies are intended to increase informal learning which focuses on the lessons that can be learned from life experiences (Marsick & Watkins, 1990). Learning in this context – without a high degree of design or structure, and where citizens reflect on their experiences in interaction with others – often increases community confidence and capacity to define its own needs and identify its own priorities (Stein, 2002).

While informal and incidental learning generally take place without much external facilitation or structure (Marsick & Watkins, 2001), PATH uses a facilitated process to engage and guide the group or community in developing their own community health impact assessment tool. This facilitated process involves two separate but related activities: the PATH process and developing the tool; and using the tool to do community health impact assessment.

The first of these, the PATH process, is the community development process that results in the creation of a community health impact assessment tool. This process begins by having community members share and reflect on their experience about what makes and keeps their community healthy. A technique of storytelling, adapted from Labonte and Feather's (1996) structured dialogue approach, is used to help generate stories about these experiences. Through the stories, community members learn about the web of socio-economic factors determining their health. Underlying this process is an assumption that people know a considerable amount about what makes them and their community healthy (Gillis, 1999; Gillis & English, 2001).

The structured dialogue method (Labonte & Feather, 1996) is then used to help community members critically reflect on the experiences that affect their health or the health of their families. Using their stories, people are asked the following questions: What did you see happening in this story? (description); Why do you think this happened? (explanation); So, what does this tell us about factors that determine health in your community? (synthesis); and, finally, Now, what can we do about it? (action). This process is based on Kolb's (1984) experiential learning cycle, which is recognized as an effective means of facilitating group learning. By sharing stories and critically reflecting on them, a space is created where community members learn with and from each other and produce shared insights. The experience creates collective knowledge that is owned by the members of the community or group (Imel & Stein, 2002). This group discussion process provides an opportunity for community members to broaden their understanding of the factors determining health, and they learn that they can take action to support health in their community (Gillis, 1999; Schneider, 1997).

Based on this broader understanding of health, community members then focus on developing a vision of what their healthy community would look like. Participants use their own words and emphasize their priorities in their vision of a healthy community. They draw on the interaction in the group and their common experiences and collective knowledge. This process helps community members learn that they can analyse their own real life problems and establish solutions that work in the context of their community (Coady, 2010).

While communities often identify similar factors that determine their health, their vision statements often reflect distinctively different priorities. For example, while increased employment was a priority and central to the visions of a healthy community in PATH I and PATH II, an increased sense of value and empowerment for women was central in the vision put forward by the women in the West Bengal village.

Following the development of a vision, community members then examine the major components of their vision and answer the following question: What would be happening in the community if the different parts of this vision were being achieved? What would this healthy community look like? The answers to these questions identify the indicators that can be sorted, prioritized, and incorporated into a systematic list of questions, which forms the community health impact assessment tool. The informal learning involved reinforces that they can identify directions for future action that can safeguard the health of their community. Information typically included in the tool is a statement of the values and principles that guided the work, a vision statement for a healthy community, a summary of key determinants of health, and a list of factors important in building and sustaining a healthy community (Mittelmark, 2001). Depending on the context, the format and presentation of the tools may vary. For example, in the development of their tools, the three communities in PATH 1 used art metaphors to complement textual representations of their culture and of their vision of a healthy community. The tool, unique to the community that produced it, is then tested, and revised if necessary, on a real or imaginary program or policy.

The second part of the facilitated process involves using the tool to do a community health impact assessment. The use of the tool requires clearly defining the policy, program, or project to be assessed, gathering a group of people to do the assessment, facilitating the use of the tool, gathering further information if necessary, and writing up summaries and developing a plan of action (PATH & NCCHPP, 2007).

The adult learning strategies incorporated in PATH are intended to stimulate informal learning in response to situations, which require action at the individual, group (community), and systems (policy) levels. Such informal learning enables people to take action related to their health at one or more or all of these levels. Consistent with these intents, project evaluations of PATH reinforce that the adult learning strategies involved strengthen the adult learning possibilities, build community identity, and stimulate a desire among individuals and groups involved to move towards constructive action on issues affecting health (Peters, 2002; Schneider, 1997). This is a point that English also makes in her discussion of health impact assessment tools.

Lessons Learned

The implementation of PATH across a variety of settings and cultures has resulted in significant lessons being learned about each of the two sets of activities involved. These lessons, described below under their corresponding headings, highlight conditions that support a community-driven health impact assessment.

The PATH Process and Developing the Tool

The experience across all contexts where PATH and community health impact assessment has been implemented is that the PATH process leading to the development of a tool is highly educational and empowering. It enables people to reflect on and to analyse their situation. They learn about the social, political, cultural, and economic factors that affect their health, and they develop a vision of a healthy community. Beginning with the telling of stories, people from very different socio-cultural contexts are able to make sense of their experiences and they learn that the determinants of their health are interconnected (English, 2000; Gillis, 1999; Gillis & English, 2001). An emphasis on networking and working within and between communities in PATH I enabled the communities involved to expand their analysis and understanding to factors influencing the health of the whole region.

Participation in the PATH process often also leads to unanticipated empowerment outcomes. For example, highlighting their cultural context, the tribal women in West Bengal cited the opportunities to have a say and to be heard as among the most important benefits of being involved in the process of community health impact assessment (Ghosh & Cameron, 2006). This is consistent with Kolb's (1984) idea that knowledge is created through the transformation of experience.

The development of the tool is always grounded in a broad vision of health, and the activities involved enable people to identify a wide range of supports and constraints to their health. In addition to knowledge about these determinants of health, the process also enables people to identify factors that they see as important priorities in their communities. For example, in generating and analysing information using the story dialogue method in PATH I, one of the communities involved recognized the need for a more holistic approach to health education. Shortly after the end of the project, they launched a health information centre and programs to address the social determinants of health in their community. Similarly, following participation in the PATH I process in West Bengal, India, village women organized a range of health awareness programs in schools and in their communities to promote healthy behaviours. They learned that they could take action related to their health.

The PATH process also builds people's capacities to engage in informed decision-making and health planning at the community level (Cameron, 2009). As people learn about the supports and challenges to healthy living, they are more able to envision the kinds of changes that can protect and improve the health of their communities. Use of the tool generates knowledge and information – both positive and negative – which can be used for decision-making, but also to raise awareness and to build a case for advocacy. For example, since its development, the Antigonish Town and County Community Health Board tool has been used by a variety of groups facing funding cuts, including the local women's centre, an affordable housing society, and a local literacy association (http://www. antigonishwomenscentre.com/reports.htm). They used the tool to estimate the impact of funding cuts to their programs and the health and well-being of the community, and to advocate for community support of their services. While not all groups that develop community health impact assessment tools have used the actual tools, they have often used the PATH process in other community endeavours. For example, through the PATH process, the women's self-help group in West Bengal identified micro-enterprise endeavours, and then lobbied to get the training they needed to set up their own micro-enterprises (Cameron, 2005). In Nova Scotia, the PATH process has been used in a variety of community-based participatory research projects, including one aimed at exploring how literacy affects peoples' health (http://www.nald.ca/ healthliteracystfx/findings.htm).

Key elements of the design of PATH also make the activities involved empowering for community members. For example, in doing community health impact assessment, local knowledge is validated – an empowering outcome for community members. Respect for the lived experience of adults is a core principle in adult education (Knowles, 1990; Lindeman, 1982). In line with these beliefs, the first-hand experience of community members is a central resource in community health impact assessment.

The PATH process also provides continuous opportunities for meaningful dialogue. Community members learn from their experiences and are able to look at both sides of an issue without conflict. From this dialogue and their reflections, they are able to realize their potential to be involved in local decision-making and to influence public policy. Because PATH builds on life experiences and values indigenous knowledge systems and oral traditions, it is a process that can be used in many cultures and contexts (Cameron, 2009). In addition to geographic communities, community health impact assessment has application in settings where policy and programs are developed or implemented, such as health care settings, non-governmental organizations (NGOs), schools, and workplaces.

The participatory process is as important as the tool developed from that process (Gillis, 1999). The participatory structure in PATH and community health impact assessment is highly inclusive and enables many voices and perspectives to be heard. In all settings, it has been important to involve people from many sectors, in order to represent the ideas and views of the community. The engagement and training of local facilitators in PATH I – who were familiar with the community, its key organizations and agencies, local leaders, and both the formal and informal channels of communication – resulted in broader community participation (English, 2000; Gillis, 1999). In PATH II the vision of a healthy community was based on the input from 57 local focus groups; in Mukutmanipur, the tool was developed by the Tourism Management Committee along with the local women's self-help group, thus ensuring that voices from a variety of sectors were heard. Participatory learning is an integral part of enabling people to establish common goals and to work together to effect social change in their communities (Vella, 2002).

The experience with PATH and community health impact assessment has also shown that there is a need to balance the process of awareness-raising among community members with the actual development of the tool. This enables them to realize the value of the process as well as the outcomes. Both of these activities are health promoting and important (Cameron, 2009). For example, in the case of the tribal community in Mukutmanipur, the processes of storytelling, visioning, and developing a list of questions for their tool enabled participants to realize all of the factors that affect their health, while the use of the tool led them to realize the potential negative effects of a proposed tourist project on village harmony, their culture, and youth. As they moved forward with an action plan for the tourist project, they put safeguards in place to mitigate these potentially negative effects. The PATH process had helped them to analyse critically their situation and to come to an understanding of factors they had previously not considered. This is essentially the learning cycle of Kolb (1984). As community members reflect on their experiences and everyday problems, they are able to translate their experience into concepts, which they use as guides for active experimentation, and the choice of new experiences and alternatives. In this way the PATH processes provide opportunities for the continuous construction of new meaning and knowledge.

The activities involved also respect community timelines and informal leadership. Although a significant time commitment from community members is required, the development of the tool is a concrete goal of the PATH process which motivates people to stay involved. While it is possible to take an existing tool and adapt it to the local context, experience shows that the *process* of creating the tool is one of community empowerment, and is every bit as valuable as the CHIAT itself (PATH, 2008). If the process of sharing stories, developing a vision of a healthy community, and understanding how determinants act together to influence health is missed, the tool may not have the same relevance to the community (Gillis & English, 2001).

Doing Community Health Impact Assessment

Doing community health impact assessment helps communities learn that they can take action related to their health and that they can be involved in developing healthy public policy. However, decision-makers need to understand the value of community input, and the process requires support from them. Moreover, the experience of implementing PATH in a variety of settings, contexts, and cultures has revealed that community health impact assessment requires support both during and following the process of creating a tool (Cameron, 2009; Gillis, 1999; Mittlemark, 2001).

Initially, the social and political environment must be favourable and supportive of community input (Mahoney, Potter, & Marsh, 2007). The earliest implementations of PATH reinforced that support from the broader systems of decision-making (e.g., health systems, municipal governments, community-based organizations) is essential, if the results of the assessment are to have an impact, and if use of the tool is to be sustained. In PATH I and II, the community partnership of local organizations, with a shared interest in the health of their communities, joined together to build the community process, to facilitate the community discussion and the development of the tool, and to support community use of the tool. This partnership continues today through the PATH Network, which continues to function as 'a network of groups and individuals, sharing ideas and resources to build healthy communities in northeastern Nova Scotia' (PATH, 2008, p. 1). Without this kind of commitment to involving citizens in health decision-making and drawing on more than a top-down approach, community health impact assessment loses much of its relevance (Gillis, 1999; Gillis & English, 2001).

This need for broad system support extends to the provision of funding to support such community-based processes that require time and administrative support so that people can develop the necessary leadership and facilitation skills (Cameron, 2009). The PATH process and community health impact assessment is acknowledged to require significant facilitation skills (Cameron, 2009; English, 2000; Gillis, 1999; Gillis & English, 2001). However, training of community facilitators in the requisite skills (i.e., small group facilitation, communication and active listening, structured dialogue, and participatory data analysis techniques) increases the potential for sustaining community participation in health decision-making, and more sustained use of community health impact assessment activity (Cameron, 2009). As well, support and resources are required to enable people to participate (e.g., travel, childcare costs) in community health impact assessment.

Finally, the development of a CHIAT is not a one-time event. Rather it is a long-term community development process focused on enabling community members to become informed about health and to influence policy. While community-driven forms of health impact assessment may be labour intensive and challenging (Mahoney, Potter, & Marsh, 2007), they offer potential as a simple, highly practical process that can enhance significantly a community's awareness and capacity to come to grips with local circumstances that need changing for better health.

As important as administrative and funding support, communities also need access to epidemiological or hard data in an understandable format so they are able to make informed decisions. Often the processes identify other information that is required to make informed decisions such as environmental impact assessment or business financial studies, depending on the context of the assessment (Cameron, 2009). For example, use of the Antigonish Town and County Community Health Board tool by a local municipal government to assess the impact of a large recreation project in 2009, revealed the need for additional information about the environmental effects of the planned development, and whether there was sufficient local support to go ahead with it.

Conclusions and Implications

Community health impact assessment brings together community development, health promotion, and adult education techniques to enable communities to learn about a broader concept of health, see their vision of a healthy community, and have a tool that they can use to plan for their future. As a values-based and community-driven form of health impact assessment, it provides a strategy for communities (and networks of organizations within them) to have an open dialogue on what it takes to make and keep a community healthy. Community health impact assessment equips communities with new knowledge and the skills to ensure that the diversity of conditions that directly affect their health and well-being are considered in the development of public policies and programs. As a strategy to support community action on health, community health impact assessment can, therefore, add significantly to institutional efforts to safeguard the health and well-being of individuals and communities.

As this chapter highlights, community health impact assessment also provides a strategy to facilitate adult and community learning related to health. It is a participatory process, called for by English in the first chapter of this book and by many of the authors in Part II, that encourages community members to have a more holistic perspective on health. It recognizes the community's knowledge in their understanding of the determinants of health and enables community members to develop strategies to develop their own healthy community. The significant learning which occurs for them in the processes of both developing and using a tool is empowering and consistent with the goals of health promotion and education. For adult and health educators and community development practitioners who strive to minimize health inequalities through the promotion of community learning and action, community health impact assessment can provide an appropriate health promotion and health education response and strategy.

REFERENCES

Barnes, R., & Scott-Samuel, A. (2000). *Health Impact Assessment (HIA): A ten-minute guide.* International Health Assessment Consortium, University of Liverpool. Retrieved 10 October 2011 from http://www.liv.ac.uk/PublicHealth/obs/publications/hia/hialeaflet3.pdf

Buchanan, D.R. (2006). A new ethic for health promotion: Reflections on philosophy of health education for the 21st century. *Health Education & Behaviour, 33*(3), 209–304. doi:10.1177/1090198105276221.

Coady, M. (2010). Community health impact assessment (CHIA): Fostering community learning and healthy public policy at the local level. In S. Brigham &

D. Plumb (Eds.), *Proceedings of the 29th Annual Conference of the Canadian Association for the Study of Adult Education*. Montreal, Quebec.

Cameron, C. (2009). Community health impact assessment: Safe-guarding community well-being. Paper presented at the International Association for Impact (IAIA) 2009 Conference. Acra, Ghana.

Cameron, C., & Ghosh, S. (2005). Empowering communities. *Health Action, 18*(8), 29–31.

English, L.M. (2000). Spiritual dimensions of informal learning. *New Directions for Adult and Continuing Education, 85:* 129–38.

Ghosh, S., & Cameron, C. (2006). *Strengthening communities through community health impact assessment.* Paper presented at the International Conference Towards Strength-Based Strategies that Work with Individuals, Groups and Communities. Hyderdad, India.

Gillis, D.E. (1997). *PATHways to building healthy communities in eastern Nova Scotia: The PATH Project resource.* Antigonish, Nova Scotia. Retrieved 6 June 2009 from http://www.antigonishwomenscentre.com/reports.htm.

Gillis, D.E. (1999). The People Assessing Their Health (PATH) project: Tools for community health impact assessment. *Canadian Journal of Public Health, 90*(1), 53–57.

Gillis, D.E., & English, L.M. (2001). Extension and health promotion: An adult learning approach. *Journal of Extension, 39*(3).

Hancock, T. (1985). Beyond health care: From public health policy to healthy public policy. *Canadian Journal of Public Health, 76*(1), 9–11.

Hancock, T., & Minkler, M. (2002). Community health assessment or healthy community assessment: Whose community? In M. Minkler (Ed.), *Community organizing and community building for health* (pp. 139–157). Piscataway, NJ: Rutgers University Press.

Imel, S., & Stein, D. (2002). Adult learning in the community: Themes and threads. *New Directions for Adult and Continuing Education, 95:* 93–97.

International Association of Impact Assessment. (2006). *Health impact assessment: International best practice principles.* Special publication series no. 5. Retrieved 10 October 2011 from http://www.iaia.org/publicdocuments/special-publications/SP5.pdf.

Kemm, J. (2001). Health impact assessment: A tool for healthy public policy. *Health Promotion International, 16*(1), 79–85.

Knowles, M. (1990). *The adult learner: A neglected species.* Houston, TX: Gulf.

Kolb, D.A. (1984). *Experiential learning.* Englewood Cliffs, NJ: Prentice Hall.

Labonte, R., & Feather, J. (1996). *Handbook on using stories in health promotion practice.* Ottawa: Health Development Division, Health Canada.

Lindeman, E.C. (1982). To put meaning into the whole of life. In R. Gross (Ed.), *Invitation to lifelong learning* (pp. 118–122). Chicago: Follett.

Mahoney, M.E., & Durham, G. (2002). *Health impact assessment: A tool for policy development in Australia*. Burwood, Australia: Deakin University. Retrieved 15 July 2009 from http://www.deakin.edu.au/hia.

Mahoney, M.E., Potter, J.L., & Marsh, R.S. (2007). Community participation in HIA: Discords in teleology and terminology. *Environmental Impact Assessment Review, 17*(3), 229–241. doi:10.1080/09581590601080953.

Marsick, V., & Watkins, K. (1990). *Informal and incidental learning in the workplace*. New York: Routledge.

Marsick, V., & Watkins, K. (2001). Informal and incidental learning. *New Directions for Adult and Continuing Education, 89*; 25–34.

Mittelmark, M. (2001). Promoting social responsibility for health: Health impact assessment and healthy public policy at the community level. *Health Promotion International, 16*(3), 269–274.

National Collaborating Centre for Healthy Public Policy. (NCCHPP). (2008). Healthy public policy: How do public policies affect health? What does research tell us? Retrieved 1 March 2010 from http://www.ccnpps.ca/548/Healthy+Public+Policy.htm.

National Collaborating Centre for Healthy Public Policy. (2009). Influencing healthy public policy with community Health Impact Assessment. Retrieved 10 October 2011 from http://www.ccnpps.ca/docs/PATH_Rapport_EN.pdf.

People Assessing Their Health Network (PATH). (2002). PATHways II: The next steps. A guide to community health impact assessment. Retrieved 8 January 2009 from http://www.ccnpps.ca/514/Publications+and+Presentations.htm.

People Assessing Their Health Network (PATH), & National Collaborating Centre on Healthy Public Policy (NCCHPP). (2007). The PATH process and community health impact assessment *(CHIA)* [brochure]. Retrieved 16 June 2009 from http://www.ccnpps.ca/514/Publications+and+Presentations.htm.

People Assessing Their Health Network (PATH), & National Collaborating Centre for Healthy Public Policy (NCCHPP). (2008). Review of documentation and learnings: People assessing their health *(PATH)* [brochure]. Retrieved November 2009 from http://www.ccnpps.ca/514/Publications+and+Presentations.htm.

Peters, N. (2002). *Applying community health impact assessment to rural community health planning: Evaluation report*. Antigonish, NS: Author. Retrieved 5 June 2009 from http://www.antigonishwomenscentre.com/reports.htm.

Schneider, R.A. (1997). *PATH project evaluation final report.* Baddeck, NS: R.M. Schneider Associates. Retrieved 5 January 2009 from http://www.antigonish womenscentre.com/reports.htm.

Simpson, K., & Freeman, R. (2004). Critical health promotion and education: A new research challenge. *Health Education Research: Theory & Practice, 19*(3), 340–348. doi: 10.1093/her/cyg049.

Stein, D.S. (2002). Creating local knowledge through learning in community: A case study. *New Directions for Adult and Continuing Education, 95:* 27–40.

St-Pierre, L. (2008). Roundtable on health impact assessment [Background paper]. Montreal: National Collaborating Centre for Healthy Public Policy. Retrieved 5 January 2011 from http://www.healthypublicpolicy.ca/en./liste resumes.aspx?sortcode=2.1.1.2&id_article=231&starting=&ending=.

Stuttaford, M., & Coe, C. (2007). The 'learning' component of participatory learning and action in health research: Reflections from a local sure start evaluation. *Qualitative Health Research, 17*(10), 135–1360. doi: 10.1177/1049732307306965.

Tones, S., & Tilford, S. (2001). *Health promotion: Effectiveness, efficiency and equity* (3d ed.). Cheltenham, UK: Nelson-Thornes.

Vella, J. (2002). *Learning to listen, learning to teach: The power of dialogue in educating adults.* San Francisco: Jossey-Bass.

Wilkinson, R.G. (1996). *Unhealthy societies: The afflictions of inequality.* London: Routledge.

Wilkinson, R.G. (2006). Politics and health inequalities. *The Lancet, 368*(9543), 1229–1230.

World Health Organization. (1986). Ottawa charter for health promotion. Retrieved 2 March 2009 from http://www.who.int/hpr/archive/docs/ottawa.html.

World Health Organization. (1997). Jakarta declaration on leading health promotion into the 21st century. Retrieved 1 October 2011 from http://www.who.int/healthpromotion/conferences/previous/jakarta/declaration/en/index.html.

World Health Organization. (2008). Closing the gap in a generation: Health equity through action on the social determinants of health. Retrieved 1 August 2010 from http://www.who.int/social determinants/thecommission/finalreport/en/index.html.

3 Community-Engaged Health Research: Communities, Scientists, and Practitioners Learning Together

LINDA ZIEGAHN

Adult educators are in a position to suggest inclusive learning models that can help health researchers, health practitioners, and members of the public at large bridge gaps between laboratory science and adoption of medical discoveries. They have a key role to play in working with communities in assessing their health needs, learning with them and teaching them about health, and involving them in research processes on matters that affect their health.

Health research is often perceived as unrelated to the day-to-day health concerns of individuals and communities, for several reasons. The first stems from health policy research findings that a good share of scientific discoveries never make it into day-to-day clinical practice or to those individuals who could most benefit. Health researchers have identified disconnects between research breakthroughs initiated in the laboratory and their progress, to human studies, to clinical practice, and eventually to adoption by the public (Michener et al., 2009; Westfall, Mold, & Fagnan, 2007; Woolf, 2008). As examples, a large-scale survey of adults living in 12 metropolitan U.S. areas revealed that only about 55 per cent of health care recommended by physicians was received by study participants (McGlynn, Asch, & Adams, 2003). Further, only about one-quarter of participants with diabetes received routine monitoring tests, individuals with hypertension received 65 per cent of recommended care, and only 38 per cent of participants had been screened for colorectal cancer, despite the demonstrated benefits of screening technologies.

From an educational perspective, these findings suggest that producers of health research and providers and recipients of health services do not share common perceptions of appropriate recommendations for care or who is qualified to create the knowledge that leads to the diffusion and adoption of advised treatments. New, more inclusive paradigms of health research are proposed in which community members inform the research process, so that values and practices around health are identified from the beginning and integrated into the formulation of research questions (Minkler & Wallerstein, 2008; Woolf, 2008; Zerhouni, 2005). These models of community-engaged research are based on philosophies of collaboration similar to those used in adult learning and are useful in explaining the formation of academic-community partnerships. However, such models seldom frame these partnerships in terms of their learning potential. This interest in community partnerships is echoed by many writers in this volume, including Moseley, Coady and Cameron, and Egan.

The second impetus for rethinking how health research is conducted is the perception by many consumers that researchers are generally isolated in academic pursuits that yield conflicting information of dubious use to routine health decision-making (Minkler & Wallerstein, 2008). The language used in research is seen as esoteric, reflective of the basic science undertaken in laboratories rather than in 'real life,' and in the linguistic codes of experts rather than in lay language. This 'expert-lay person' dichotomy is further fuelled by the perception that power dynamics have favoured the academic researcher's role, whereas the public's stake in research is often perceived as limited to that of potential participants in clinical trials and eventual consumers of the treatments and interventions resulting from health research. Complicating this 'us-them' view, particularly from the perspective of under-represented and minority populations, is the long history of the unauthorized involvement of participants in research in which clinical trial participants from marginalized communities were appallingly ill-treated, such as those African Americans not informed of advances in treatment of syphilis in the decades-long Tuskegee experiments (Thomas & Quinn, 2001). The learning environment is thus compromised by feelings of confusion and disinterest among health consumers around the ultimate benefit of health research, and, more alarming, feelings of betrayal and distrust of both research and researchers.

Among the people who are the ultimate beneficiaries of advances in health research, the poor and marginalized suffer disproportionately from disease, both physical and mental, and limited access to care (Marmot, 2005). Communities that are under-represented in medical research tend to differ from those groups that historically have been well represented in clinical trials – educated whites, higher in literacy and income (Giuliano et al., 2000). The individuals and communities that might benefit most from advances in health research – those living in poverty or in minority linguistic and cultural communities – are also most likely to be excluded from opportunities to shape research initiatives and to benefit from research which reflects their culture and life circumstances as well as their medical status. Thus the power dimension of potential learning models that promote collaboration among all parties is critical.

The challenge for communities and health professionals – a category which may include researchers as well as doctors, nurses, and other clinicians working directly with patients – is *learning* how to reconceptualize health research in a new climate of shared power and expertise. This chapter will explore: how the addition of adult learning theories to models of community-engaged research from the field of health can set the scene for collaborative learning and research to improve health care for all through discussion of stakeholder interests; a hypothetical example of a health partnership from the perspectives of researchers/clinicians, and community members; a comparison of models of community-engaged health research and complementary adult learning theories; and suggested areas for learning for all stakeholders in academic-community health partnerships.

What Is Community-Engaged Research, Who Is Involved, and Why?

Community-engaged research is a process in which academic researchers, clinicians, and members of communities defined by geographic proximity, similar interests, or situations jointly define, conduct, and evaluate research that is rooted in mutual interest, needs, and respect (Fawcett et al., 1995; Jones & Wells, 2007; Minkler & Wallerstein, 2008). All must learn enough about each other's health expertise and lifeworlds so that they can develop shared goals, language, and processes for embarking upon research that improves health. Researchers from outside the community may have scientific knowledge, but not fully appreciate the local context of a given health problem, just as community members not trained in research will have many questions about the nuances of research methods and study design (CTSI & UCSF, 2009). For example, a top official of the Urban League of Greater Pittsburgh, Lee J. Hipps, described the experience of working with University of Pittsburg cardiologists on a community-based study to identify risk factors associated with heart disease. They were able to significantly increase recruitment of African Americans in the study because they listened to community requests for assistance with health screenings and other interventions; or, as Hipps explained, 'Rather than saying "We [the research community] want something from you," we went to the community asking, "What can we do for you?"' (Bonetta, 2008, pp. 4–5).

There are a number of potential stakeholders most directly involved in the project of community-engaged health research in the context of poor and/or marginalized communities. The first of these is *individuals within communities* that are under-represented in health research due to ethnicity, race, economic status, gender, sexual orientation, or other marginalizing factors. These communities can include different racial and ethnic groups, women, children, adolescents, people in poverty, rural dwellers, the elderly, and lesbian, gay, bisexual, transgender, and questioning (LGBTQ) individuals. Reasons for their lack of participation may vary, but the most common are geographic isolation, a history of discrimination, low literacy, and/or linguistic and cultural differences. Individuals involved in community-engaged research may be leaders or other representatives of community-based organizations such as neighborhood associations, community health clinics, or service organizations; grass-roots advocates for particular communities; or health care workers who grapple with the effects of unsuccessful health care interventions.

The second group of stakeholders includes a broad range of health professionals from both the clinical practice and research sectors. First are *clinicians* – specifically the physicians, nurses, physicians' assistants, and other professionals who work regularly with marginalized communities in community clinics, private practice, non-profit organizations, or public health agencies. These individuals experience first-hand the bureaucratic, financial, cultural, and linguistic hurdles faced by people trying to gain access to regular and effective health care. They are also aware of the routine health problems which plague particular communities. In addition, *community outreach workers* and *health educators* frequently get involved as partners in health research, and are often asked to assume the role of broker between academic investigators and communities. Health outreach workers and educators represent a broad range of experience and training backgrounds, including adult education.

This second group also includes *researchers*, or investigators, who typically initiate proposals for research ideas to be sent to a variety of federal, state, and private foundations for funding consideration. Lead researchers on projects generally assume the title of Principal Investigator (P.I.), and are responsible for the initial design, operation, and evaluation of the eventual research project. P.I.s are typically college or university faculty members (MDs or PhDs), public health or social service professionals, physicians in managed care networks or private practice, graduate students in science, or medical students. In community-based research projects, P.I.s can also come from partner community organizations. Finally, *clinical research coordinators (CRCs)* are responsible for managing recruitment and retention of clinical trial participants, ensuring that participants are treated in accordance with ethical research guidelines, and monitoring research protocols and procedures. Most CRCs have been trained as nurses or physician assistants, or are graduates of bachelor or masters of science programs.

All share a stake in the enterprise of maintaining good health and wellness, regardless of socio-economic, education, or legal status, and all are potentially engaged in learning to communicate across long-standing barriers separating health scientists from the general public. The range of scientific projects around which research can be conducted is vast, but centres generally on either biomedical research focused on evaluation of new treatments, or on health services research on the design, delivery, and evaluation of health programs.

The learning that occurs in health research collaborations can shift between several contexts, including the research laboratory, clinical practice, and/or community-based entities. Suggested below are two typical scenarios:

An Example of Community-Engaged Research from the Perspective of the Researcher or Clinician

Dr Jackson, an assistant professor in pediatrics at a large university, has been conducting research on the effectiveness of glucose monitoring technologies and their impact on the management of Type 1 diabetes in children. She is aware that this question is particularly relevant to the children of Mexican immigrants living in the large urban area in which her practice is located. She would like to recruit children and their families into a clinical trial in which where she can further study this phenomenon. However, as a junior researcher, she is unsure how to go about recruiting participants. She is aware that simply posting flyers will not necessarily be sufficient to attract those most suitable for her study. She also knows that as an outsider to Mexican culture and a non-Spanish speaker, she may be less likely to convince anyone to sign up for the study. Her clinical research coordinator, Rogelio Gonzalez, a nurse of Puerto Rican descent, is most anxious to help, but he also has many questions about how to get the word out. He is aware that immigrant communities are wary of outsiders from large institutions coming to tell them they have programs that will be of benefit, only to learn that the group that benefits most is the institution, not the individual or the community.

An Example of Community-Engaged Research from the Perspective of Community Members

The leadership of the El Centro community centre is increasingly disturbed at the high rate of diabetes in both the parents and children who frequent their programs. The neighbourhood in which they live, often referred to as 'Little Mexico,' is characterized by gang violence, high unemployment, and, above all, isolation from the larger metropolitan area. Kids have few places in which to play, after-school programs are almost nonexistent, and diets are characterized by food high in carbohydrates and fats from the one major supermarket in the area. Many of the clinic clients are in the United States illegally, and live in fear of being found out by immigration authorities. However, the community has many strengths, including a fledgling parents' group at the local middle school interested in fighting against gang activity, and a small clinic staffed by a committed, if overworked, staff. El Centro leaders are aware that they live not far from a major university medical centre, but do not really know what goes on there. Occasionally they hear stories from people who have been patients at the university hospital and experienced serious problems trying to cross language and cultural barriers around their care – a problem not that different from other attempts to communicate with 'the system.' El Centro staff are also wary of the 'experts' who came to collect information on problems in the past, then left and were never heard from again.

These stories from two differing perspectives share common dynamics of a lack of familiarity and distrust, but also reflect interest in learning how to improve the dismal health status of underserved communities. Scenarios such as these can lead community members, scientists, and clinicians to pose a number of questions around potentials for partnership, as illustrated below. In order to better understand how the field of health frames research involving all stakeholders, it is helpful to look at recent conceptual trends in health-based community engagement and in learning models from the field of adult education.

Models of Community-Engaged Research from Health

Community-engaged research models from the field of health reflect recent national policies aimed at moving basic scientific discoveries into the realm of actual practice and adoption (Bonetta, 2008; Woolf, 2008: Zerhouni, 2005). Health policy-makers are increasingly interested in ensuring that research be connected not only to the realm of the laboratory, but also to the communities in which medical innovations are eventually expected to be used. Researchers should learn to listen to the ultimate consumers of scientific discoveries from the starting point of research question formulation, rather than only at the end point of recruitment for clinical trials. *Learning* how to engage communities in this relatively new environment of shared power and expertise involves the inclusion of previously ignored participants such as communities and clinicians. Key concepts in new, more collaborative models of health research are bidirectional learning and communication (Zerhouni, 2005) through which the local knowledge of communities is on par with the scientific knowledge of academic researchers. A number of 'best practices' for community engagement in service of these concepts emerged from a recent series of United States Center for Disease Control-sponsored workshops: move the frame of traditional biomedical research from an 'us' to a 'we' orientation, putting community interests first; broaden the definition of community to include community clinicians and public health workers as well as academics; acknowledge historical mistakes and be creative in engaging the community in the research agenda; share power, 'work yourself out of a job, but leave a trace'; level the playing field through development of a common language around research and include community partners in funding; include community members in internal reviews of research proposals; train community researchers; and disseminate findings back to community partners and community clinicians (Cook & Community Engagement Steering Committee, 2009).

Bolstering this emphasis on collaborative academic-community research are several interconnected frameworks on engaging underserved communities in identifying research topics, conducting research, and disseminating findings around mutually defined health research outcomes:

community-based participatory research (CBPR), asset-based community building, and culturally competent health research. While these models do not necessarily address the learning that occurs in research that includes community members, health professionals, and academic researchers, they are useful in spelling out the accompanying processes and participants.

While adult educators have long advocated for community-based learning around social justice goals (Freire, 1970; Horton, 1990; Locke, 1938), a more recent approach from the field of health is community-based participatory research (CBPR). Probably the best known model of community-engaged health research, CBPR shares common ancestors with the adult education field such as critical theorists Paulo Freire (1970), John Gaventa (1999), and Budd Hall (1992). Some of the key principles of CBPR include: (a) building on strengths and resources within the community; (b) facilitating collaborative, equitable partnerships that foster power-sharing among all stakeholders; (c) promoting co-learning and capacity building around the construction of local health belief theories; (d) striving for balance between research and action for the benefit of all partners; (e) recognizing the multiple determinants of health and disease that affect local communities; (f) dissemination of findings and knowledge to all partners involved; and (g) a commitment to sustainability and long-term collaboration around research (Israel, Schulz, Parker, & Becker, 2001; Minkler & Wallerstein, 2008).

The primary contribution of the asset-based model to the project of community-engaged research is acknowledging and building upon the 'strong neighborhood-rooted traditions of community organizing, community economic development and neighborhood planning' (Kretzmann & McKnight, 1997, p. 9) of lower-income and marginalized communities. This is in contrast to the competing model of many social service agencies, including health agencies, in which poor communities are viewed as an endless reservoir of 'needs' which require intervention by these same agencies. As an example, community pediatricians at the University of California Davis used an asset-based approach to improve child health in a Sacramento neighborhood (Pan, Littlefield, Valladolid, Tapping, & West, 2005). They started by assessing their own assets as physicians, then completing an asset map of the community by interviewing key stakeholders and surveying the physical and economic assets of community associations. Emerging from these joint academic-community data collection activities were specific events and interventions that helped to reduce the incidence of particular health problems affecting children in the neighborhood.

A central focus of community-engaged research is increasing responsiveness to the health concerns of poor and minority racial and ethnic communities. Consequently, the concept of cultural competence is essential not only to researchers' efforts to understand different beliefs around causes of disease, effective treatments, and who in the community is qualified to give medical advice, but also to envision how communities, medical practitioners, and researchers can collaborate to improve health care and its delivery. Goals of culturally competent care (and by extension, research) include 'creat[ing] a healthcare system and workforce that are capable of delivering the highest-quality care to every patient regardless of race, ethnicity, culture, or language proficiency' (Betancourt et al., 2005, p. 500). Cultural competence and community-engaged research share emphases on developmental processes for both individuals and organizations that evolve over time (Cross, Bazron, Dennis, & Isaacs, 1989) and on the reciprocal transfer of knowledge and skills (Taylor & Brown, 1997). At the stage of cultural proficiency, individuals and organizations are able to establish and maintain networks of diverse groups beyond 'traditional' health care boundaries, with the goal of 'eliminat[ing] racial and ethnic disparities in health and mental health' (National Center for Cultural Competence, 2007).

Cultural competence models are criticized for a number of reasons, such as treating culture as a variable, inadvertently setting up a climate in which a patient's culture is blamed for failure to adapt to the medical system, focusing more on cultural differences than similarities and thereby obscuring structural power imbalances, and failing to recognize biomedicine as a cultural system itself (Carpenter-Song, Nordquest Schwallie, & Longhofer, 2007). Ironically, these are the very failures that health professionals sought to mitigate by revisioning health care as a process that rejected the belief that 'one size fit all.' Nonetheless, the inclusionary goals of the cultural competence model hold true for both health care delivery and research.

Learning Models from Adult Education Relevant to Community-Engaged Research

The field of adult education provides several models that can help us understand how learning occurs in the context of community-engaged health research in which multiple stakeholders collaborate around goals of both individual and systemic transformation and change. Community-engaged research calls for bidirectional communication and equalized relationships between researchers, practitioners, and community members, as demonstrated in the health-related community-engaged research models discussed above. Learning within the framework of community-engaged research calls for a recognition of additional attributes of the research environment: specifically, the contexts in which research is developed and conducted, the life experiences of stakeholders, and a vision of the inclusive social change that can result from collaborative process. Experiential learning and transformational learning are useful heuristics in this exploration, and they are at the heart of many chapters in this book, especially in Chovanec and Johnson (chapter 8).

In her review of current conceptions of experiential learning, Fenwick (2000) identified a number of learning perspectives in terms of their utility for understanding cognition and learning. From the perspective of community-engaged research, the constructivist, situative, and resistance approaches – overlapping concepts, each with a distinct focus – can lead us to a better understanding of the learning that takes place among participants in community-engaged research projects. In constructivism, 'a learner is believed to construct, through reflection, a personal understanding of relevant structures of meaning derived from his or her action in the world' (Fenwick, p. 248). In community-engaged research, participants learn through paying attention to the differentials of status, areas of knowledge and expertise, and arenas in which change can be affected. For example, in the Hmong community, traditional healers can help researchers to understand how Hmong participants in a cancer research project might construct the root causes and treatment options for cancer. In turn, researchers can bring to an academic-community research partnership knowledge of effective cancer treatments from the perspective of Western medicine. Through an iterative, collaborative research process grounded in reflection, they can redefine approaches to better cancer care and management.

Situative perspectives, including situated cognition and Wenger's (1998) communities of practice (CoP) model, allow for the simultaneous linking of knowing, learning, and doing in contexts which may differ substantially. For example, university-based community meetings which 'include' community members in discussions around health are very different from community meetings in which researchers are invited to share not only knowledge, but also processes of agenda initiation, meeting facilitation, and outcome identification. In CoPs, learners interact around a common goal through joint enterprise, such as a community-engaged research project, and through a shared repertoire of language and resources. Established research norms are challenged, and a particular research problem, such as the high incidence of diabetes in El Centro, becomes the context in which learning occurs. Participants 'invent' practice situated in everyday existence, improvisation, coordination, and interactions.

In situative perspectives, competence is not the provenance of just one individual, but rather of a variety of stakeholders who come together through shared practice. To return to the El Centro case, who are the experts on the best strategies to combat diabetes? Those who have the biomedical knowledge, or those who have personal experience with the disease and are faced with its management within ever-changing socio-economic and cultural environments? In CoPs, new ideas emerge from the disparate work and community contexts in which stakeholders practise. While Lynam (2009), in her review of critical pedagogy in the field of nursing, questioned whether biomedical perspectives can be anything but 'objective ... remov[ing] disease from its social context' (p. 51), the premise of community-engaged research is that more inclusive and productive bidirectional communication between the laboratory, the clinic, and communities can break down the long-held assumption that biomedical and health research must by necessity exist apart from ultimate beneficiaries.

Important to the understanding of the learning that occurs within contexts characterized by power imbalances is the notion of resistance, categorized by Fenwick (2000) as a type of experiential learning. Resistance is rooted in the politics and cultural dualisms influencing ideas about who produces knowledge and how knowledge is exchanged. The academic environment of community-engaged research is coloured by memories of the hegemonic role of science in improving the health of some but not necessarily all, and by the present-day geographic realities of universities often situated in the midst of urban poverty. Quigley's (1987, 1997) exploration of why potential literacy learners resisted schooling, and subsequently basic education programs, is relevant to the case of community-engaged research. He makes the point that learning, objective knowledge, and education were not necessarily opposed. Rather, low-literate learners resisted pressures to relinquish personal rights to live otherwise and to escape oppressive and hypocritical institutional learning environments. Similarly, in community-engaged research, members of underserved communities who feel alienated by unapproachable health workers, physicians, and unresponsive bureaucracies may opt out of the 'system' – not because they do not value learning about healthy behaviours. Rather, they may feel that the loss of control and sense of self-efficacy around their own mental and physical health is too great a price to pay for what little they receive. A critical element of community-engaged research is thus learning from resistance – from marginalized community members as well as health professionals and researchers.

Transformational learning is based on revision of the underlying premises of beliefs and perspectives, through a process of critical reflection (Mezirow, 1991). Points of view, informed by moral-ethical, psychological, and epistemic perspectives (Mezirow, 2000), ultimately shape meaning schemes on a subliminal level around cause and effect relationships, sequences of events, or portrayals of others. In the case of community-engaged research, how do African Americans, for example, view the intent of health researchers asking for clinical trial participants? Or, how do researchers characterize the knowledge base and interest of members from a range of communities in the conduct of basic health research? Unless individuals engage in critical reflection, the tendency would be for health professionals and community members alike to pursue their usual habits in thinking about the other, about motivations, and about consequences of actions.

Within the framework of transformational learning and critical reflection, the process of learning about the other is particularly relevant to the philosophy and methods connected with community-engaged research. It is often assumed that there is a direct path between awareness of the differences between peoples and groups and a subsequent transformation in expectations about how best to provide responsive health care (Blackford & Street, 2002; Lynam, 2009). Critical reflection can provide the bridge between awareness and transformation of meaning schemes. In a study of the types of reflection that characterized graduate student online postings around cultural difference in a class on inclusive community building, Ziegahn (2005) identified six approaches important to adoption of more critical perspectives: linking personal positions to specific cases of inequity; embracing negative emotions that arise from reflection on the complexities surrounding cultural and social justice issues; questioning long-standing personal prejudices; reframing underlying premises and personal beliefs around culture and equity; suspending judgment and attempting to understand the perspective of others; and linking new experiences to previously learned habits of critical reflection.

These findings have relevance for the scientists, health practitioners, or community members who may feel they are encountering a new culture when they cross traditional boundaries separating academe from the life-world, and seek alternative ways of reflecting upon the status quo.

In critically reflective learning, the emotional or affective aspects of learning are equally as important as the cognitive dimensions of learning that evolves around long-standing attitudes and beliefs (Boud, Cohen, & Walker, 1993; Kovan & Dirkx, 2003; Ziegahn, 2005). Both a critical stance and attention to emotional cues are particularly important to all stakeholders embarking on collaborative community-academic health research. Reframing past traumatic interactions with health institutions so that future learning can occur in a positive environment character-ized by healthy self-esteem, trust, and support necessitates an attention to the emotions accompanying the stories of community member con-tact with health systems and research.

Learning for Stakeholders in Community-Engaged Research

How can all stakeholders in health research ensure that medical findings are translated into community practice and actually result in improved health for all? First, it is important to recognize the many differences which arise when stakeholders collaborate to improve individual and community health – differences in culture; political and economic power; resources to effect change; and, significantly, strengths or assets. In particular, while community members may appear to operate from a disadvantaged position in partnerships with academic researchers, they bring to the table considerable strengths, particularly around perspec-tives on local health issues and disparities.

Learning to recognize strengths is a process that has the potential to change attitudes, knowledge, and skills for all participants in the context of community-academic health partnerships. Table 3.1 suggests areas of learning which may serve the interests of community members, research-ers and health professionals, or all groups.

Additionally, it may be useful for community members considering involvement in community-engaged research to think about these questions:

- Why should we be interested in research, particularly since many of our concerns relate primarily to our need for direct services?
- How can we interest researchers in the health problems that affect our community?

Table 3.1. Learning in Community-Engaged Research

Areas of learning	For community members	For researchers and health professionals
How to approach academic researchers about local health concerns	X	
Key problem identification, design, conduct, and evaluation stages of biomedical and/or health services research	X	
The administrative context of health research, in terms of safeguards for human participants, funding cycles, proposal writing, and project deliverables	X	
Basic proposal writing components	X	
How to view health researchers as potential allies in improving community health	X	
Local and regional demographics on health disparities; which communities suffer disproportionately from particular health conditions	X	X
How to present basic scientific studies to communities in lay terms		X
Identifying and gaining access to community organizations interested in partnering around a mutually identified research topic		X
Temporary suspension of the 'habits' of thinking about expertise as belonging only to scientists; inclusion of community members as possessors of expertise around health issues	X	X
Listening to the varied interests of community members about not only health research but also health in general		X
Training approaches for involving community members in community-engaged research	X	X
Theory and practical steps (e.g., data collection instruments) in community-engaged research models, such as CPBR or asset-based community development	X	X
The potential roles for community members, health practitioners, and researchers in the various phases of community-engaged research	X	X
The ethical context of health research and how it affects communities and stakeholder relationships	X	X
Effective communication strategies in discussions of community interests, historical inequities, and collaborative health research from the perspectives of community members and organizers, health practitioners, and academic researchers	X	X
Establishing long-term community-academic partnerships	X	X

- How can we receive training in how to assess our own health issues, together with academic partners?
- Where should we look for funding for health research ideas?
- What instruments would be most appropriate to evaluate the effectiveness of some of our health care programs?
- How can we be assured that researchers will understand and appreciate the particular cultures of our communities?
- Will we be considered equal partners?

Similarly, researchers and other health professionals might bear these questions in mind when weighing the value of participating in community-engaged research:

- What are the questions of community members around my field of interest? What impact does this particular disease have on them?
- How can I set up a relationship with community groups interested in my research?
- Where and how would I look to draw a sample of community participants for a research study?
- How can I get feedback on my research proposal from the community?
- How will I know if my needs assessment or intervention strategies are linguistically and culturally appropriate?
- Where would I look to assess the impact of particular health interventions in an evaluation study?
- How do I train community members in aspects of research design in ways that reflect respect for their knowledge as well?
- How can I build relationships with community partners that endure beyond our initial research effort?

In summary, the field of adult education has much to add to health-based theories of community-engaged research. Community members, clinicians, and researchers have the opportunity to form communities of practice grounded in bidirectional communication between all parties. Critical to the work of these collaborative entities, in which participants negotiate research priorities and procedures, assign responsibilities, and hypothesize possible impact and results, is recognition of the transformative potential of learning that validates the importance of 'disorienting dilemmas' (Mezirow, 1991) and resistance as motivators for change. Critical reflection on areas of difference – through questioning sources of disorientation and resistance, reframing past experiences with medical institutions and health resources, suspending judgments around who 'should' have knowledge about health and what kind of knowledge is valid – is essential for stakeholders stimulated by the prospects of health research that reflects the interest, energies, and goals of all those seeking improvement in our collective health.

REFERENCES

Betancourt, J.R., Green, A.R., Carrillo, J.E., & Park, E.R. (2005). Cultural competence and healthcare disparities: Key perspectives and trends. *Health Affairs 24*, 499–505.

Blackford, J., & Street, A. (2002). Cultural conflict: The impact of Western feminism(s) on nurses caring for women of non-English speaking backgrounds. *Journal of Clinical Nursing, 11*, 664–671.

Bonetta, L. (2008). Engaging communities. NCRR Reporter: Critical Resources for Research. (winter/spring), 12 (1), 4–8.

Boud, D., Cohen, R., & Walker, D. (1993). *Using experience for learning.* Buckingham, UK: Society for Research into Higher Education & Open University Press.

Carpenter-Song, E.A., Nordquest Schwallie, M., & Longhofer, J. (2007). Cultural competence re-examined: Critique and directions for the future. *Psychiatric Services, 58, 1362–1365.*

Clinical and Translational Science Institute (CTSI), & UCSF. (2009). Collaboration with UCSF researchers: A guide for community organizations and agencies. Retrieved 5 July 2009 from the UCSF Clinical and Translational Science Website: http://ctsi.ucsf.edu/research/community-manuals/.

Cook J., & Community Engagement Steering Committee. (2009). *Researchers and their communities: The challenge of meaningful community engagement.* Washington, DC: Clinical and Translational Science Award Consortium, Center for Disease Control and Prevention, Association for Prevention Teaching and Research Cooperative Agreement No. U50/CCU300860.

Cross, T., Bazron, B., Dennis, K., & Isaacs, M. (1989). Towards a culturally competent system of care. *National Technical Assistance Center for Children's Mental Health.* Vol. 1. Washington, DC: Georgetown University Child Development Center.

Fawcett, S.B., et al. (1995). Using empowerment theory in collaborative partnerships for community health and development. *American Journal of Community Psychology, 23,* 677–697.

Fenwick, T. (2000). Expanding conceptions of experiential learning: A review of the five contemporary perspectives on cognition. *Adult Education Quarterly, 50*(4), 243–272.

Freire, P. (1970). *Pedagogy of the oppressed.* New York: Seabury Press.

Gaventa, J. (1999). Citizen knowledge, citizen competence, and democracy building. In S. Elkin & J. Soltan (Eds.), *Citizen competence and democratic institutions* (pp. 49–66). State College: Pennsylvania State University Press.

Giuliano, A., et al. (2000). Participation of minorities in cancer research: The influence of structural, cultural, and linguistic factors. *Annals of Epidemiology, 10*(8), S22–S34.

Hall, B. (1992). From margins to center? The development and purpose of participatory research. *American Sociologist, 23(4),* 15–28.

Horton, M. (1990). *The long haul.* New York: Anchor Press.

Israel, B.A., Schulz, A.J., Parker, E.A., & Becker, A.B. (2001). Community-based participatory research: Policy recommendations for promoting a partnership approach in health research. *Education for Health, 14*(2), 182–197.

Jones L., & Wells K. (2007). Strategies for academic and clinician engagement in community-participatory partnered research. *JAMA, 297,* 407–410.

Kovan, J., & Dirkx, J. (2003). 'Being called awake': The role of transformative learning in the lives of environmental activists. *Adult Education Quarterly, 53,* 99–118.

Kretzmann, J., & McKnight, J. (1997). *Building communities from the inside out: A path towards finding and mobilizing a community's assets.* Evanston, IL: Northwestern University, Asset-Based Community Development Institute, Institute for Policy Research.

Locke, A. (1938). *Negro needs as adult education opportunities,* pp. 254–261. Findings of the First Annual Conference on Adult Education and the Negro, held at Hampton Institute, Virginia, 20–22 October 1938 under the auspices of the AAAE, the Extension Department of Hampton Institute, and the Associates in Negro Folk Education.

Lynam, M. (2009). Reflecting on issues of enacting a critical pedagogy in nursing. *Journal of Transformative Education, 7*(1), 44–64.

Marmot, M. (2005). Social determinants of health inequalities. *The Lancet, 365,* 1099–1104.

McGlynn, E.A., et al. (2003). The quality of health care delivered to adults in the United States. *New England Journal of Medicine, 348,* 2635–2645.

Mezirow, J. (1991). *Transformative dimensions of adult learning.* San Francisco: Jossey-Bass.

Mezirow, J. (2000). *Learning as transformation: Critical perspectives on a theory in progress.* San Francisco: Jossey-Bass.

Michener, L., Scutchfield, F., Aguilar-Gaxiola, S., Cook, J., Strelnick, A., Ziegahn, L., et al. (2009). Clinical and translational science awards and community engagement: Now is the time to mainstream prevention into the nation's health research agenda. *American Journal of Preventive Medicine, 37*(5), 464–467.

Minkler, M., & Wallerstein, N. (Eds.). (2008). *Community-based participatory research for health: From process to outcomes* (2d ed.). San Francisco: Jossey-Bass.

National Center for Cultural Competence. (2007). Homepage. Retrieved 6 June 2009 from http://www11.georgetown.edu/research/gucchd/NCCC/foundations/frameworks.html.

Pan, R.J., Littlefield, D., Valladolid, S.G., Tapping, P.J., & West, D.C. (2005). Building healthier communities for children and families: Applying asset-based community development to community pediatrics. *Pediatrics, 115*(4), 1185–1187.

Quigley, B.A. (1987). Learning to work with them: Analyzing non-participation in adult basic education through resistance theory. *Adult Literacy and Basic Education, 11*(2), 63–70.

Quigley, B.A. (1997). *Rethinking literacy education: The critical need for practice-based change.* San Francisco: Jossey-Bass.

Taylor, T., & Brown, M. (1997). Developing educational and service leadership roles. Paper presented at the Faculty of Professional Development and Mentoring, University of Oklahoma Health Sciences Center, Oklahoma City.

Thomas, S.B., & Quinn, S.C. (2001). Light on the shadow of the syphilis study at Tuskegee. *Health Promotion Practice, 1,* 234–237.

Wenger, E. (1998). *Communities of practice: Learning, meaning, and identity.* New York: Cambridge University Press.

Westfall, J.M., Mold, J., & Fagnan, L. (2007). Practice-based research – 'blue highways' on the NIH roadmap. *JAMA, 297(4),* 403–406.

Woolf, S.H. (2008). The meaning of translational research and why it matters. *JAMA 299*(2), 211–213.

Zerhouni, E. (2005). Translational and clinical science – time for a new vision. *New England Journal of Medicine, 353,* 1621–1623.

Ziegahn, L. (2005). Critical reflection on cultural difference in the computer conference. *Adult Education Quarterly, 56*(1), 39–64.

4 Advocacy, Care, Promotion, and Research: Adult Educators Working with the Community for Health

JOHN P. EGAN

This chapter examines various developments in Canadian health care, particularly how health care in Canada has evolved to meet the needs of community and how community has been involved in changing health care. In particular, the role of adult education – teaching, learning, co-researching, and activism – is highlighted, since adult education principles have often been an integral part of changing policies and practices. This chapter examines adult education's role in working with the community formally and informally to create change and to strengthen the health of communities.

Health Promotion as Adult Education

Although developments with respect to health in Canada have oftentimes been driven by adult education, in many instances the actors involved might not explicitly describe themselves as educators. Yet they often describe in detail evidence of effective andragogy (Knowles, 1988). This group of educators includes allied health professionals (such as nurse, nutritionists, occupational therapists, dentists, and physicians) and community members (promoting health and wellness, as well as agitating for access to care and services – both locally and at the policy level). Whether conducted in the context of health services, community outreach, or social marketing, health promotion has, at its core, a focus on teaching and learning.

There are a number of important developments related directly to health and learning identified in this chapter. But it bears reminding that it has been developments in other fields that have done much to improve the length and quality of life for Canadians. Creating social distance between people and their waste products – sewage drains and enclosed plumbing, in other words – has dramatically reduced the spread of diseases transmitted via contact with human waste. Centralized plumbing has meant people have easy access to potable water, which can also be used for wash one's self, clothes, and home more often and more thoroughly – all of which reduces the transmission of disease. The development of secure, safe water and waste systems have changed human history. These structural changes, though not in strictest terms health services, have nonetheless greatly reduced the frequency and severity of illness. Building and maintaining such infrastructure requires stable, systemic governance: the benefits of such systems serve as a reminder that individuals and communities are responsible for their health and for ensuring their needs are met by those involved in service provision. With the advent of mass infrastructure, there has been an increase in people's desire to gain control over their own health and their management of it. This is a theme echoed in many chapters in this book, especially by Atleo (chapter 6), who focuses on how First Nations in this country have struggled to manage their health. This community dimension involves adult education practices of dialogue and teamwork and contributes to the long-term health of the population.

In less than half a century, health care in Canada has been revolutionized. Until the mid-twentieth century, seeking and receiving (or not) health care was considered a private matter. Today Canada's (ostensibly) public health care system has standards of care, supported by structures at government, private sector, and community levels, which are among the best in the world. In fact, many Canadians view access to health care as both a human right and civic entitlement. They want to be participants in change and to have their voices heard – both key adult education principles.

While there is inherent complexity in terms of the challenges to provide effective care to over 30 million people, health care in Canada is a remarkably simple institution in terms of how it operates. Despite being a quasi-public (i.e., government) institution, throughout its history our health care system has developed according to the needs of community, writ large and small. As our understanding of health broadens, ownership of keeping Canadians healthy is evolving beyond a traditional medical treatment model (diagnosis, treatment, recovery of health) to one of holistic population health. For this to function well, community members need to be an integral part of the decisions and policies that affect them.

International

Efforts in Canada to promote health have long been entwined with those of the international community. In 1986 the World Health Organization (WHO) convened its first international conference on health promotion in Ottawa. From that meeting a charter of health promotion principles (now referred to as the Ottawa Charter) was produced. Subsequently other charters have been proposed, but some 25 years later the Ottawa Charter (WHO, 1986) remains a document that informs health promotion strategies worldwide.

The Charter defines health promotion as 'the process of enabling people to increase control over, and to improve, their health' (p. 1), and identifies nine fundamental conditions to achieve this: peace, shelter, education, food, income, a stable ecosystem, sustainable resources, social justice, and equity. These, described as the foundation of good health, are collectively known as wellness, and they are remarkably similar to the goals that most adult educators working in the community want to achieve. The degree to which each of these is fulfilled significantly impacts one's capacity for wellness; where several are absent, one's capacity to maintain wellness is more greatly impeded. However, even if some – or all – of these fundamentals are missing, effective health promotion is possible, if nonetheless more challenging.

These represent an intersection of ecology (characteristics of the physical world in which we live), society (our communities and related structures, including culture), and our values (how we make meaning of the world, how we assess our actions as ethical or not). Whether in a rural setting where literacy may be basic and infrastructure poor, or in an urban setting where literacy is the norm but social justice is absent, in both contexts – in any context – deficiencies in these conditions lead to vulnerability to disease and death. When health professionals and community members become engaged in a collective process of health promotion, enabled by an adult education approach, more of these issues can be addressed.

The Ottawa Charter also identifies with six means of action (or components) for developing effective health promotion initiatives. These include:

- support at the policy level (including stable financial support);
- sustainable development (ecological, social, and economic);
- strengthening community action (to foster empowerment);

- individual skill development (through lifelong learning);
- reorienting health services to a health promotion (rather than diagnose and treat) model; and
- equality for all (particularly for girls and women) (WHO, 1986).

This health promotion model recognizes the importance of engaged citizenry and active involvement in learning about our health and our care. It does not suffice to leave to officials, governments, and health care professionals all decisions regarding wellness and the provision of health services. Whereas their expertise is essential, it can well be supplemented by adult education expertise in community involvement and both informal and nonformal educational practices.

It is important to remember that the Charter (WHO, 1986) is a statement of principles. It does not offer instruction on how existing health services can be reorganized to work within a population health approach – or how to create new entirely new services to replace existing ones. This central challenge – realigning or replacing health services so they reflect a substantive commitment to population health – is in many ways the core narrative of health care in Canada since the Second World War. In this sense, adult educators can work with health professionals to bring these principles to life.

Health Promotion

A geographic orientation to health services delivery often works better at an administrative level than it does for communities, particularly stigmatized or marginalized communities. We have a surfeit of data that show how certain diseases and conditions are more prevalent (the percentage of persons in a community with a disease or condition) in specific communities than in the general population. Examples of this include: (a) late onset (Type 2) diabetes among new Canadian women (PHAC, 2009); (b) malnutrition among off-reserve Aboriginal children (McIntyre, Connor, & Warren, 2000); (c) obesity among impoverished persons (Public Health Agency of Canada, 2009). Each of these communities is unique; each has its own values and local practices. Generic health promotion strategies for these conditions have not mitigated them. Implementing local initiatives based on a population health approach, however, can.

According to Kindig and Stoddart (2003), a population health model for health services delivery takes into account 'the health outcomes of a group of individuals, including the distribution of such outcomes within the group' (p. 380). Integral to a population health approach is understanding of the (social) determinants of health – different aspects of lived experience that affect how healthy individuals are; which should be taken into account in determining service provision, strategy, and resource allocation. Social determinants of health reposition the conditions described in the Ottawa Charter (WHO, 1986) as requisite for health promotion to occur, particularly in terms of barriers to health. Race, ethnicity, and gender are determinants of health because racism and sexism are barriers to social justice and equity. Adult educators' knowledge of these factors that affect health make them especially helpful in enabling communities to acknowledge them also, and to work with legislators, community members, and disadvantaged populations to address them.

Yet, the shift towards population health does not refute the geographic, medicalized distribution model; the costs to do so, in terms of building wholly new structures and systems, would be exorbitant. It instead adapts current services based on a more nuanced understanding of how certain medical conditions manifest themselves – particularly the circumstances of those having developed (or are vulnerable to developing) that condition. Adult educators can be very helpful here in facilitating discussions in the community, working with community health boards to find workable solutions, and in negotiating conflicts over core areas.

At an immediate level, much of this work involves shifting the discourse around health promotion – quite literally a task that adult educators are often well prepared for. For persons whose command of a majority language is not strong, materials and services are offered in their primary languages. Thus the commonplace strategy of producing health promotion flyers in multiple languages is a population health strategy, though at a relatively passive and superficial level. Conversely, finding service providers who speak community languages – or persons who can readily translate what can be dense medical and scientific language for someone visiting a health care provider – is a more active and substantive strategy. If literacy is an issue, simplified majority language materials with cartoon graphics are also used. These strategies are versions of those used by any adult community educators working in minority communities: outreach services as a form of community education. If the physical location of health programs and services cannot be moved, outreach strategies – communication, transportation, locally hosted clinic, or support groups – are often used by adult educators to facilitate access to care.

The advent of grass-roots social justice movements – women, Aboriginal persons, francophones, queers, persons with disabilities, and new Canadians, among others – has brought a shift towards population health: service adaptation to the person requiring services, rather than that person adapting him/herself to services created with service provider needs at the fore. It is from adult community education – often informal – that the impetus to shift service delivery has come. Educating one's peers, educating service providers, even educating public officials are all examples of this. Community education is the theme of many chapters in this text, including Moseley's (chapter 10) on public health nursing.

Geography versus Population

Perhaps the most important development in Canadian health policy in the last 20 years has been a shift in how health service delivery is organized and evaluated. As discussed above, the traditional health services delivery model is structured wholly in geographic terms: services have been organized based on where people live. Thus, in areas of greater population concentration there have been more services (and more provider options); in areas with relatively sparse populations there have been fewer services, with little or no specialized care provided locally. Perhaps, in a basic way, this makes sense: supply and demand. But in a country where thousands live in rural settings hundreds (or even thousands) of kilometres from a major urban centre, this skews access to health services. For persons with no access to general practitioners in their communities, travel to another community is required. As a result, many simply do not seek care, except when already significantly ill or injured. Despite initiatives designed to mitigate the dearth of services in rural Canada, living in a rural setting remains a social determinant of health – and a focus among community educators seeking to improve access to care in their rural communities. Adult educators with expertise in working in rural communities can help communities identify the ways in which they are affected by their geographical location and help them address issues such as inadequacies in transportation to access medical and other services.

Within large urban centres health services can become stratified: impoverished persons often have to wait longer to access the few health care providers willing to see them. As a result, many rely on hospital emergency rooms for their primary care. In addition to poverty, Aboriginal persons and new Canadians often find it hard to secure a general practitioner, which leaves drop-in clinics and hospital emergency rooms as their venues for primary care. Ostensibly, while everyone living in a major Canadian city should have similar access to care, in practice, persons vulnerable to discrimination have less. Again, adult educators with expertise with disadvantaged populations can work with them to garner public support, organize for change, and have an effect on public policy.

Population Health in Canada

When adult educators become involved in creating change they need to ask some fundamental questions. Does it make sense to have health services wholly based on population density? Or should some services be positioned closer to communities – populations, in health services parlance. These community-focused questions are within the realm of adult education work, and, though often contentious, need to be addressed.

The success of many communities in agitating for improved access to care across Canada is due to the groundwork laid by the women's health movement, which drew greatly on adult education principles. While many conflate reproductive rights (contraceptives and abortion) with women's health activism, in reality this movement's scope has been – and remains – much larger. At a very basic level, much of the movement's focus has been to challenge structural biases that leave women more vulnerable with respect to some conditions (such as heart disease), or offer scant services for conditions that only affect women (such as cervical or ovarian cancers).

In seeking better diagnosis, treatment, and care in these areas, the women's health movement's larger agenda has been about making the linkages between women's experiences seeking care and systemic gender bias – sexism – in society. It is in the area of making linkages, drawing connections, and raising consciousness that adult education has contributed to this movement. By initially creating alternative structures that operated at the grass-roots community level, women stepped out of a system that served them badly, equipped themselves with the knowledge required to make informed choices, and challenged caregivers to provide services on their terms. Today there is a rich patient-centred, self-advocacy-oriented culture in terms of health services delivery (in most instances; mental health services and addictions services are notable exceptions) – largely attributable to the women's health movement. This input into delivery of services is concomitant with growing community awareness of its rights and responsibilities for health. Women's health activists also took on a patriarchal health services culture, where men were in charge (physicians) and women were servants (nurses). When women demanded more information about their conditions they challenged the notion that physicians decided what care was provided. Concomitantly, more women pursued careers as physicians and health researchers.

Today women play leadership roles at every level of health service administration, delivery, and research. They have served as ministers of health at the provincial, territorial, and federal levels. Currently the deans of medicine at the Universities of Toronto, Ottawa, and Western Ontario are all women.

If women first catalyzed a shift towards patient-centred care (and therefore towards population health), other communities quickly followed their example. And it is women who are leading the movement in professions such as nursing to more community involvement in decision-making, health care governance, and in the promotion of education on the broader determinants of health such as the quality of the environment. Community involvement and participation is a core adult education principle, and the success of the women's movement is a prime example of how this participation can result in effective and long-term change.

HIV/AIDS

There are other examples of how vulnerable communities have changed health services in Canada through the use of adult education principles such as relationship building and public awareness. The story of Acquired Immune Deficiency Syndrome (AIDS) in Canada offers us a unique opportunity to see how health promotion with respect to a new condition evolves over the condition's entire 'lifespan.' Most of the primary causes of debilitating illness in Canada (including heart disease, cancer, arthritis, diabetes) were identified in humans hundreds of years ago: in contrast, AIDS was first diagnosed in Canada in 1981, which means it had to have appeared here within the previous three to 10 years. In the first years of the AIDS epidemic in Canada, the condition was not well understood; thus, we can also see how health promotion evolved as our understanding of AIDS evolved – from ignorance, to identification of cause, and to the advent of largely effective treatment. In chapter 5 of this book, Ntseane and Chilisa discuss AIDS from an African perspective; yet many of the issues are similar.

Now into its third decade, over 65,000 persons have been diagnosed as having been infected with the human immunodeficiency virus (HIV) since widespread testing began in 1985 (PHAC 2009). However, the number of persons living with HIV today could be much higher, since persons who are newly infectious are usually both asymptomatic and hyperinfectious. To date, over 12,000 AIDS deaths have been recorded in Canada, about half of whom were queer men (PHAC 2009).

The impact of HIV/AIDS among queer men has been particularly staggering, especially in Vancouver, Toronto, and Montréal; in this respect, vulnerability based on homophobia has been the social determinant of health. Subsequently, AIDS has spread beyond queer men, with injection drug users, persons receiving contaminated blood products (prior to 1985), and women all significantly impacted. Yet the grass-roots response to HIV/AIDS has been robust and effective – ahead, in many ways, of that of public health. In the early days of the epidemic, beginning in 1981, groups of gay men in cities across Canada began organizing themselves to provide information and support. AIDS Vancouver's founding members included physicians, gay rights activists, and a Vancouver city councillor. Very quickly these men began disseminating prevention information, despite the fact that scientists had not yet identified HIV as the cause of AIDS. In fact, it was these men at AIDS Vancouver who first proposed that gay men should abstain from blood and other human tissue donations, since it seemed likely that whatever caused AIDS was transmissible through this mode. This case highlights the adult education strategies of public campaigns, teaching vulnerable populations through informal means and reliance on the strength of the community.

And while much of the focus of grass-roots HIV/AIDS work continues to prioritize queer men, as the epidemic broadened to include other vulnerable communities (particularly injection drug users), a harm-reduction approach implemented by queer men was adapted to other contexts. Often these contexts have differed, as have the techniques proffered to reduce harm, but the overarching principles have remained the same: peers educating one another, to reduce risk and remain well. This is an informal adult education strategy that appears to have worked well in this community. The initial promotion of condom use during anal or vaginal intercourse by anyone vulnerable to HIV infection via sexual intercourse subsequently evolved to the promotion of the use of new syringes by injection drug users. The core principle is the same: if stopping a behaviour that creates risk is not tenable, find strategies to mitigate risk. Effective condom use and not sharing syringes are both robust ways to reduce the potential for HIV transmission. As a form of health promotion, harm reduction is taught formally through health services and community services. But much harm reduction education is peer-based and informal. In fact, many harm reduction strategies develop within communities and are then disseminated more widely via health and community services. It was several years after local AIDS groups in Vancouver were promoting condoms as harm reduction that public health officials in British Columbia integrated condom use into their HIV education programs. Community educators led the way and other professionals followed, in this instance.

Many nascent AIDS activists had little experience in social justice work. But queer men learned much from their lesbian peers, whose experience in the women's health movement proved invaluable. There was no shortage of knowledge and skills among queer men back then; combined with the community education experience of queer women, a rapid community response was mounted. The challenge was an adult education one: to acknowledge indigenous knowledge and integrate it into the public discourse.

Just as women had infiltrated health services in search of better care, AIDS activists began agitating for similar change from government. They advocated for better care in hospitals, acceptance of same-sex partners as family members, and for access to new, even experimental treatments. Later they fought for changes in how health research was conducted. They demanded community advisory committees be created to inform research processes, then they endeavoured to have community members as research team members. Eventually they secured places on grant reviewing committees in research funding bodies, to ensure funds went to studies that reflected community priorities and needs. Over time, many community-based AIDS organizations began doing their own community-based research. Today community-based research is an acknowledged, if not wholly embraced, legitimate health research paradigm. This development is part of a long line of community agitation for a say in its own health care. Thus, adult community education related to health in Canada has evolved: from advocacy, to health promotion, and through the health research enterprise. Community engagement in research that directly affects its health is discussed by Ziegahn in chapter 3.

Community

Our health care systems in Canada reflect Canadian society and our social union. As acceptance of Canada's diversity has grown, a shift towards health service and insurance systems that adapt to communities' needs (rather than communities adapting themselves to service structures that create barriers to access) has emerged. Concomitantly, our shared aspiration for a publicly administered health insurance régime has faced its own challenges – most notably fiscal viability while maintaining timely access to effective care.

The evolution of health services in Canada has been driven by community – and actioned often via community education and activism. Looking forward, the onus remains on community to ensure the Canadian approach is sustainable and ensures the health and wellness of all Canadians. Still, health services continue to work within a treatment model rather than prevention. Few would argue against the value of preventative services – services to maintain wellness rather than treat illness – but no such shift seems to be in the offing. This is perhaps because our systems already struggle with the provision of care for the current disease burden in Canada, leaving little bandwidth for expanded preventative services. Regardless, whether oriented towards treatment or prevention, just as the onus remains on community to ensure our entitlements to health and wellness, so too will the teaching and learning of adults remain at the fore.

REFERENCES

Deber, R. (2003). Health care reform: Lessons from Canada. American Journal of Public Health, 93(1), 20–24.
Health BC. Media site: Provincial median wait times. Accessed 18 September 2009 from http://www.health.gov.bc.ca/cpa/mediasite/waitlist/median.html).
Health Canada. (2005). Canada Health Act, Frequently asked questions. Accessed 18 November 2009 from http://www.hc-sc.gc.ca/hcs-sss/mediassur/res/faq-eng.php.
Kindig D., & Stoddart G.L. (2003). What is population health? American Journal of Public Health. 93(3), 380–383.
Knowles, M. (1988). The modern practice of adult education: From pedagogy to andragogy. Boston: Cambridge Press.

Lacoursière, J., Provencher, J., & Vaugeois, D. (2001). Canada-Québec. Montréal: Septentrion.

McIntyre L., Connor S.K., & Warren, C.J. (2000). Child hunger in Canada: Results of the 1994 National Longitudinal Survey of Children and Youth. Journal of the Canadian Medical Association, 163(8), 961–965.

Public Health Agency of Canada. (2009). Backgrounder: What Is AIDS? Accessed 20 September 2009 from http://www.phac-aspc.gc.ca/aids-sida/publication/mon-surv/index-eng.php.

United Nations Development Program. (2009). Human development report 2007/2008: Fighting climate change: Human solidarity in a divided world. New York: Palgrave Macmillan.

World Health Organization. (1986). Ottawa Charter for Health Promotion. Geneva: WHO.

5 Indigenous Knowledge, HIV, and AIDS Education and Research: Implications for Health Educators

PEGGY GABO NTSEANE
AND BAGELE CHILISA

HIV and AIDS research in Africa continues to demonstrate that the health of an individual is a complex issue involving the social, cultural, spiritual, physical, economic, and political aspects of African communities' collective lives. To be successful in this complex context of HIV/AIDS, those working in the area of health and HIV/AIDS education need to research, train, and educate themselves and others on local and indigenous knowledge attributes. Although there are many health educators who work in the area of HIV/AIDS, we see the primary beneficiaries of the content of this chapter as nurses, peer educators, public health activists, social workers, community members, researchers, schools, community-based organizations, and researchers implementing HIV prevention programs, especially those working in non-Western contexts such as those in Africa. In this chapter we discuss the role of indigenous knowledge in mitigating the HIV scourge, African Indigenous learning values and methods that inform care and support for the sick, and how these can be used to communicate HIV prevention strategies. We argue that the ethics of care for the sick informed by the *ubuntu/botho* ('I am we') philosophy can assist health educators, researchers, and policy-makers to appreciate the role of indigenous knowledge (IK) in the training of HIV/AIDS health educators. This concern for learning around this disease is shared by Egan in chapter 4.

Competing Knowledge Systems

Our starting point is that the failure of health educators to affect and change risky health practices and behaviours is partially explained by the coexistence of two knowledge systems, one dominant and the other peripheral. It is common sense that the current knowledge society features domination over who can know, who can create knowledge, and whose knowledge can be bought. For instance, there is evidence of unjustified and counterproductive tendency in intellectual circles to denigrate and dismiss as irrelevant and primitive indigenous knowledge. Chilisa (2005) has argued, for instance, that what we know about HIV/AIDS and pre-vention education, the information communication strategies and inter-ventions to halt the spread of HIV in Botswana, is largely influenced by the dominant First World epistemological perspectives that ignore indig-enous ways of perceiving reality. She argues that our failure to work with the framework and language of the researched means that life and death matters are either not understood or take a long time before they are understood. In addition the emergence of two competitive knowledge systems that are antagonistic to one another delays progress in combat-ing the spread of HIV/AIDS.

Elsewhere, Chilisa (2005) has demonstrated the difference between two competing knowledge systems on HIV/AIDS among residents of Botswana: one based on research participants' ways of knowing, and the other based on the researcher's knowledge and categories of analy-sis. The names and understandings given to HIV in Botswana differed depending on the context of illness. If it affected the middle aged and elderly, HIV/AIDS was called *Boswagadi*. In Tswana culture, anyone who sleeps with a widow or widower is afflicted by this incurable disease. For the majority of the young, AIDS is *Molelo wa Badimo* (fire caused by the ancestral spirits); for others, AIDS is *Boloi* (witchcraft). For Christians (Dube, 2003) 'AIDS is the Fire that is described in the Bible Chapter of Revelations, nobody can stop it' (p. 25). The people's naming is embed-ded in their perception of reality. In their world of reality, things don't just happen. There is always a cause. This cause-effect relationship is informed by careful observation that includes the supernatural, such as ancestral spirits or experience.

From the people's observation, those who died from HIV/AIDS had relationships with widows or widowers thus, the name 'Boswagadi.' For the young, a distinct observation was the appearance of herpes, *Molelo wa Badimo* (fire caused by the ancestral spirits), for herpes does look like a burn. Closely connected to this 'meaning making' is also the people's perception of health. For the Botswana and most African societies, ill-ness is associated with unhealthy relations with the family, the wider com-munity, the land, or the ancestral spirits (Dube, 2003).

Similarly, modes of transmission of HIV/AIDS derive from social rela-tions aimed at, among other things, maintaining healthy relations with the family, the community, the ancestral spirits, and the environment in general. In a study on the impact of HIV/AIDS on the University of Botswana (Chilisa, Bennel, & Hyde, 2001), focus group interviews with students identified the following as modes of spreading the HIV/AIDS virus: (a) caregiver practices – not using hand gloves, as this might mean the caregiver is not showing love to the patient; (b) the practice of *seya ntlong* (wife inheritance); in the Botswana culture the wife marries the family, thus the family has the responsibility to help raise her children; (c) unequal power relations between men and women, because as decision-makers men have the final say in sexual matters; and (d) religion, for example, in terms of church attitudes towards the use of condoms that give power to men to insist on unprotected sex.

Ideally, these ways of knowing should form the basis for understanding peoples' perceptions of realities and informing education, communication, and information strategies on the prevention of HIV/AIDS. For us, the researchers, these were treated as separate from the universal definition and modes of HIV/AIDS transmission perceived as the sole indicators of what counts as knowledge about HIV/AIDS. As Western-educated people who use Western-defined categories of analysis, we were not in a position to acknowledge the explanations of other realities.

Dismissing these perceived realities has resulted in a dichotomy of knowledge where the researched refer to 'their knowledge' (the researchers are mainly from the First World or educated in Western ways) and 'our knowledge' (the researched people's knowledge).

It is clear that when people articulated their understanding of HIV/AIDS based on their life experiences and perceptions of reality, Western researchers that included trained health educators who work in African contexts labelled that misunderstanding as awkward, a misconception, or as cultural ignorance. This is not surprising because these researchers and health educators often operate within the dominant HIV/AIDS language. Given what we know, we can suggest that health educators need to ask themselves the following questions: How is a given illness socially constructed? What are the indigenous names given to an illness? What are the indigenous perceived cures for the illness? What are the communities' constructions of cause of illness?

The Role of Indigenous Knowledge in HIV
Prevention, Education, and Research

Indigenous knowledge is used synonymously with traditional and local knowledge to differentiate the knowledge developed by a given social group or community from the knowledge generated from the Western academy and its institutions (Greiner, 2003). Dei et al. (2002), in reference to Africa, note that indigenousness may be defined as knowledge consciousness arising locally and in association with long-term occupancy of a place. Indigenousness refers to the traditional norms, social values, and mental constructs that guide, organize, and regulate African ways of living in making sense of the world.

Indigenous knowledge plays an important role in the articulation of indigenous health practices and research methodologies. Indigenous knowledge's role in framing postcolonial-indigenous health and research methodologies can be summarised as follows:

1 Indigenous knowledge is embodied in languages, proverbs and idioms, legends, folktales, stories, songs, cultural experiences of the formerly colonized and historically oppressed, and knowledge symbolized in cultural artefacts such as sculpture, weaving, painting and music, dance, rituals and ceremonies such as weddings and worshipping. Instead of relying on written literature, which is often written from the Euro-American perspective, the above sources assist in giving space and voice to non-Western indigenous ways of learning.

2 Indigenous languages and knowledge systems can enable the researcher to bring new topics, themes, processes, and categories of analysis and modes of reporting and dissemination of information not easily obtainable through conventional health knowledge, practices, and research methods. For example, the use of the Setswana cultural proverb '*botlhale jwa phala botswa phalaneng*' (meaning that young people are more knowledgeable than their parents) can be used to solicit effective HIV/AIDS education and prevention methods and messages from the youth that can then be used by peer educators in their context.

3 Indigenous knowledge can be used to enable health educators and researchers to unveil knowledge that was previously ignored, due to imperialism and colonization.

4 Health educators and researchers can draw from indigenous knowledge systems to theorize about communication strategies and methods and research processes from the perspective of the cultures and values of formerly colonized and those historically marginalized, either because of their race, ethnicity, age, gender, ableness, or religion.

5 Indigenous knowledge-driven health policies, practices, and research methodologies can enable reclamation of cultural or traditional

heritage, a decolonization of the captive and colonized mind and thought, protection against further colonization, exploitation, and appropriation of indigenous knowledge, and a validation of indigenous practices and world views.
6 Indigenous knowledge can open a space for collaboration between health educators and communities in the process of health care.

What follows is a demonstration of how researchers are invoking the Bantu people of southern Africa's abadage *Nthu, Nthu ne bathu* to debate the ethics of care in the context of the HIV epidemic.

Nthu, Nthu ne bathu: Implications for HIV Care and Support

Among the Bantu people of southern Africa one of the views of being is reflected in the expression '*nthu, nthu ne banwe*' *(Ikalanaga/Shona* version), which can be translated roughly as 'I am we; I am because we are; we are because I am' (Goduka, 2000): a person is through others. Communality, collectivity, social justice, human unity, and pluralism are implicit in this principle. The principle is in direct contrast to the Eurocentric view of humanity – 'I think, therefore, I am' – expressed by Descartes. The latter, Goduka observes, expresses a concept of self that is individually defined and 'is in tune with a monolithic and one-dimensional construction of humanity' (p. 29). In the principle of 'I am because we are,' the group's needs take priority over the individual without necessarily undermining the individual's independence.

The 'I' 'We' Obligation versus the 'I' 'You': Implications for HIV Disclosure

Jensen (2007) has argued that health practitioners, development workers, policy-makers, and researchers have at times adopted the individualistic approach to the construction of knowledge and its application. In Botswana, the UNAIDS/WHO Policy Statement on HIV Testing is an example of a unidimensional construction of humanity where the rights of the individual take precedence over that of the community (Jensen). According to the policy, the conditions under which people undergo HIV testing must be anchored in a human rights approach which protects their human rights and pays due respect to ethical principles. In practice, this has meant that the HIV testing results can be disclosed to a second party only with the permission and consent of the person affected except in cases where the individual is a minor. The policy is based on the Western medicine principle of individual confidentiality. According to this principle, doctors may not reveal what they learn about the patient without the patient's concern except to other health practitioners where it is necessary. In the Western model, individual confidentiality is necessary in building trust between the physician and the patient. The practice is in direct contrast with the practices of traditional doctors whose practice is informed by the *botho/ubuntu* 'I am we.' Among the Bantu people doctors do not practise the Western principle of individual confidentiality (Ndebele, Mfuso-Bengo, & Masiye, 2008). In traditional medicine practice, the patient visits the traditional doctor in the company of immediate family and relatives. Those who accompany the patient for consultation with the traditional doctor have a duty to report to extended family members inquiring about the health of the patient. The end result has been that while the Western medicine principle of confidentiality would not permit disclosure of a diagnosis, the traditional doctor's diagnosis is communicated to the immediate and extended family members. Under the circumstances, caregivers are more likely to rely on what they are told by the traditional doctors.

What happens when all a caregiver knows about the patient is what they have been told by the traditional doctor? What happens when a patient cannot share with the caregivers a diagnosis from Western-based medical doctors? Ndebele et al. (2008) observe that the chances of infecting caregivers or spouse may be increased in cases of patients who choose not to inform their relatives. They also note that the concept does not work well for drug adherence given that spouses and family members play an important role in promoting drug adherence. The family plays an important role in care and treatment decisions and can only do so if informed about the condition and how serious it is. As well, individual medical confidentiality does not work well with botho/ubuntu, which emphasises family, community sharing, and solving life problems together. Finally, Ndebele et al. note that illness is viewed in a holistic manner. Bantu healers look at both the biological and social consequences and address the two sides when administering treatment (p. 337). Insights from an ethical approach informed by the African Bantu *abadage* 'I am because we are' is a clear testimony of the value of indigenous knowledge in the construction of strategies for HIV prevention education.

African Indigenous Ways of Learning

The IK approach to HIV/AIDS prevention delivery, quality care to the infected, and efforts to mitigate the impact of this disease has implications for teaching and learning in the African context. In this section we share the Indigenous Knowledge ways of learning from an African context, namely Botswana, which could be adapted for HIV/AIDS education and prevention. These include the use of common understandings: namely, cultural institutions, proverbs, spirituality, participatory approaches to learning, and experiential learning.

Cultural Initiation Institutions

As a transmitter of accepted values, knowledge, skills, and moral codes, including sex education, the African culture, like all cultures, has undoubtedly ensured that what is accepted is known and passed on from generation to generation through indigenous knowledge systems. In the Botswana context, an important cultural institution that helped in the teaching and learning in all areas of life, including health and in particular sexual behaviour for young people, is the initiation schools, called *Bogwera* for young men and *Bojale* for young women. According to the literature (Khathide, 2003; Ntseane, 2006), young men and women were, among other things, taught sex education, including how to relate to people of the opposite sex, and, in some tribes, how to have sex by simulation. Penetration was firmly forbidden until marriage. Unfortunately, for many years most ethnic groups stopped practising this because when missionaries came to preach the Gospel in Africa, they did away with many cultural institutions even though most of them were good, as they maintained the moral fibre of society. As Khathide (2003) observed, the problem was that missionaries did not come up with an effective replacement. In resistance, most African cultures adopted what Khathide calls 'the conspiracy of silence' (p. 2). For example, in Botswana, talking about sex in public is considered taboo. In fact, parents are ashamed to talk about sex to their children because marital partners themselves are ashamed to talk about sex to one another. The challenge for health educators working on HIV/AIDS in cultural contexts like this is to break the silence about sexuality, especially in the home.

In Botswana, cultural leaders have started to revive these cultural training institutions such as *Bogwera* (circumcision) and *bojale* (initiation) as community-based training for young men and women. We believe that this is one IK avenue that can be used by health educators working in this context. We believe that IK and local knowledge can become part of the solution in arresting the spread of HIV/AIDS and in providing quality care, but this requires change of attitude, training, and education on the part of health educators globally.

Proverbs

The use of proverbs in the Botswana IK system is another way of constructing and acquiring knowledge that could be used in HIV/AIDS prevention education. In the Botswana cultural context, proverbs are used as common understandings of key values, knowledge, wisdom, skills, and morals that have to be passed on from generation to generation. The following are some of the proverbs that could be used to enhance HIV/AIDS prevention education.

- *Mafoko a Kgotla a mantle otlhe* means that everyone has to participate in decision-making processes that affect all. This proverb can be used in HIV/AIDS prevention education as a way of encouraging participation and individual responsibility to the prevention, support, and care in the era of HIV/AIDS.
- *Dilo makwati di tsewa mogo ba bangwe* means that we can learn from other people's experiences. Again this is something that can be used to encourage the adoption of other knowledge systems about fatal diseases such as HIV.
- *Ngwana ga a tolelwe popakwana* means that there are do's and don'ts or taboos in the care of young children. This proverb is usually used to prevent the newborn baby and the mother from infections. As a traditional health prevention value, it can be used to encourage consistent use of HIV prevention efforts as well as HIV/AIDS therapy.
- *Morogo wa ngwana ga o selwe ditlhokwa* tells us not to throw away weeds found in a child's vegetable harvest. This proverb could be used to encourage adults and health practitioners to appreciate that children can also contribute to the fight against HIV infection. Through this proverb it is believed in this culture that children's ideas or understandings could be new perspectives and solutions for the ever-changing societal problems.

We believe that cultural common understandings such as these are critical if we are to change the mindset of both health educators and researchers towards other ways of knowledge construction and sexual behavioural change.

Spirituality

Spirituality is another African IK knowledge acquisition avenue. The following dialogue (Ntseane, 2004) for community HIV/AIDS education prevention material helps illustrate how the African cultural understanding of spirituality can be related to HIV/AIDS education and prevention.

CASE STUDY 1: A conversation about HIV/AIDS in a Banyana community

MAMA-T: I hear your daughter is back from work because of ill health. What is the problem?

FRIEND: How can I know? These children are not like us who share everything, including health problems. All I know is that she is coughing and she has lost a lot of weight. It has taken too long. I am even thinking maybe it is this fashionable disease, AIDS.

MAMA-T: With swollen legs, I also suspect Boswagadi, the incurable disease. I don't know how my child could have had sex. As a young girl she attended Sunday school and she receives the Holy Communion or bread of Christ. So she knows that sex before marriage is a NO! NO!

FRIEND: Take her to the *Sangoma* (spiritual healer). Maybe your family's ancestral spirits are not happy with something and they are passing the bad omen on to the child.

MAMA-T: You are right. It is high time the family knew the problem. I was disappointed with the response from the nurse at the clinic, who said, 'The patient will tell you when she is ready.'

FRIEND: What? So they are encouraging our children to keep secrets? That is not good. Don't they know that in our culture if one is sick they whole family is sick.

This case suggests some critical areas for consideration by health educators working with HIV/AIDS in this context:

- In the church, sex before marriage is a 'shame' to the family.
- Individuals are responsible for one another's health.
- In the African culture, the living and the dead are connected, and spirits of deceased ancestors watch over us.
- Young people are not to ignore parental advice or be rejected by the church.

This section has demonstrated that in this African context, spiritual needs are also important for the body. Given that spirituality as practised in the church connects individuals to Christ and God, this can be used to provide comfort to people living with HIV and AIDS, thus helping them cope with feelings of isolation and stigma. The African culture's value of the connection between spirits of the ancestors can be used as a coping strategy.

Participatory Approaches

Participatory approaches are among the most successful counselling methods used to convey AIDS' messages, especially in oral societies. According to Dube (2003), participatory approaches include drawing, storytelling, demonstration, talking, songs, music, poems, rhymes, active listening, role play, field visits, cartoons, creative visualization, observation, and games. As Africans ourselves, we know that the methods of storytelling and group discussions are more powerful than simply providing information. Storytelling of the text and of the life of listeners or readers can serve to break the silence and facilitate hearing each other out. For instance, African stories, songs, and poems told to children in the era of HIV/AIDS can and do focus on current concerns including HIV/AIDS. The question is, are health educators and researchers working in this context listening and benefitting from this rich knowledge? We argue that it is the responsibility of the health educator and HIV/AIDS experts in particular to bring African cultural stories and HIV/AIDS together. Case 2, an extract from the Community HIV/Education material (Ntseane, 2004) for village leaders in Botswana, illustrates our point.

CASE STUDY 2: A story about a traditional doctor and an incurable disease
   (Ntseane, 2004)
FACILITATOR (FAMILY WELFARE EDUCATOR): Let us share what we know about the Matwetwe (traditional doctor). This is how the magic stick works. You ask for it if you have something to say, then you talk holding it and pass it on to the other person if you are done.
MS NINA: He is good as a diviner and herbalist.
MAMA-DO: When I said I did not trust modern medicine, I was referred to him by the modern doctors.
RADAO: He has told me that his herbs do not cure AIDS just like ARV's but I prefer his herbs.
FACILITATOR: Why do you prefer his herbs?

RADAO: It is not really his herbs but how he treats his patients. He has been my
  doctor since I was three years old. He knows my whole family. So we don't
  just *talk* about this depressing disease.
MS-NINA: Yes, he counsels me in other areas such as marriage, sibling issues, and
  so on.
MAMA-DO: His patients can consult with him at any time (night and day).
MR. KAT: Furthermore, payment is chicken, cow, anything – even free treatment
  is available.
SADI: The good thing about this Matwetwe is that whatever he does to the
  patient is explained and done in the presence of some key family members.

We hope Case 2, above, will help the reader to realise that in the African
context, the 'We' is critical. The traditional doctor has embraced it in
his dealings with patients, and the patients appreciate the fact that the
health and/or healing of an individual is a collective process. Being
accessible and understanding even in a context of HIV/AIDS encourages the search for healing.

Unfortunately, the involvement of traditional doctors in HIV/AIDS
prevention education and research has been marginalized if not disre-
garded. In fact, their efforts to help their people understand the HIV
epidemic have been dismissed as irrelevant and superstitious. Ignoring
these influential, cheap, and accessible traditional health educators is
unfortunate.

Experiential Learning

The final IK method of teaching and learning for HIV/AIDS prevention
is experiential learning. In this context, experiential learning is understood as a collaborative approach where health educators, researchers,
and learners are seen as equals. The involvement of people living with
HIV and AIDS can inform any articulation of IK that seeks to combat
HIV/AIDS. First, we believe that HIV/AIDS educators should be proactive and creative on how best to seek new methods for prevention and
care in specific contexts.

Second, we believe that through experiential learning, health educators can collaborate or even co-teach with colleagues of other speciali-
ties, as well as invite traditional health trainers from the community to
address particular areas of the epidemic. For example, sociologists can
be very critical when it comes to a social analysis of HIV socio-cultural,
infection-driving factors. Experiential learning is important because any

HIV/AIDS prevention model must be located in its specific context. As Jorgensen (2005) observes, 'competence is not merely that a person masters a professional area, but also that the person can apply professional knowledge in relation to the requirements inherent in a situation ... uncertain and unpredictable' (p. 4).

Challenges of IK in Health

We use this section to respond to the question of whether IK and local knowledge can become part of the solution in redressing the spread of HIV/AIDS and in providing quality care. We argue that the answer is yes. However, as African scholars, educators, and researchers who have worked with communities including people living with HIV and AIDS, we use this section to highlight major IK challenges.

IK is not static. Indigenous knowledge keeps changing with time and generation. This is so because it is contextually based on experiences that differ – for example, current experiences of adults versus experiences of adolescents with HIV/AIDS concerning the causes of HIV/AIDS. For the adults it is caused by *Boswagadi* (observation that those infected had sexual relations with widows who did not go through proper cleansing after losing a spouse); for the young it is caused by *molelo wa badimo* (fire from ancestral spirits) or herpes. Related to this is the fact that it is not possible to give standard knowledge. There is need for target-specific HIV/AIDS information.

Documentation. Continuous documentation is going to be a challenge because IK is always evolving. This is because African IK is cyclical compared to Western knowledge which is cumulative. Furthermore, HIV/AIDS health educators will have to be creative in finding resources given that a direct link between IK and HIV/AIDS is a subject that has been locally researched but yet does not feature in most HIV/AIDS library collections. Related to this challenge is the cost of finding willing people to provide IK information.

IK health knowledge validation. Given that knowledge validation in the health context is based on both change and benefit to society and not on disharmony and conflict with local knowledge, the challenge is that this might contrast with validation in other contexts. For example, where validity is brought by health practitioners' conformity to writing for journals, this knowledge might not even reach the community. This is a challenge because experiential knowledge is usually used immediately to bring about change.

Even with these challenges, we still argue that learning is fundamentally social because as Hensechel (1999) observed, knowledge depends on engagement. Health educators in the HIV/AIDS era have to be both qualified and competent in the role of reducing HIV infection. Competence comes later (after qualification) as health practitioners gain experience in a social environment for the development of their skill.

Conclusion

In this chapter we have argued for the integration of knowledge systems by health educators and researchers working in HIV/AIDS. In fact, they themselves should also be products of integrated and interactive learning informed by both indigenous and dominant world views about health and health systems. For them to be competent, they have to learn from other experts including those living with HIV and AIDS, families, and communities of practice. The chapter also concludes that health educators in the African context have an added responsibility of breaking the silence in sexual matters in order to successfully engage Africans in the reduction if not the elimination of HIV/AIDS infections. Finally, we believe that health educators who employ some of the IK frameworks and methods found in previously marginalized cultural contexts will be effective in reducing the spread of HIV/AIDS as well as in providing quality care.

REFERENCES

Chilisa B. (2005). Educational research within postcolonial Africa: A critique of HIV/AIDS research in Botswana. *International Journal of Qualitative Studies, 18*(6), 659–684.
Chilisa, B. (with P. Bennel & K. Hyde). (2001). *The impact of HIV/AIDS on the University of Botswana: Developing a comprehensive strategic response, knowledge and research.* Serial no 45. London: Department for International Development.
Dei, G., Hall, B., & Rosenberg, D. (2002.). *Indigenous knowledge in global contexts: Multiple readings of our world.* Toronto: University of Toronto Press.
Dube, M.W. (Ed.). (2003). *HIV/AIDS and the curriculum: Methods of integrating HIV/AIDS in theological programmes.* Geneva: WCC Publications.

Goduka I.N. (2000). African/indigenous philosophies: Legitimizing spiritu-
ally centered wisdoms within the academy. In P. Higgs, N.C.G. Vakalisa, T.V.
Mda, & N.T Assie-Lumumba (Eds.), *African voices in education* (pp. 63–83).
Lansdowne, South Africa: Juta.

Grenier, L. (2003). *Working with indigenous researchers: A guide for researchers.*
International Development Research Centre. Ottawa: www.idrc.ca/
openebooks/847-3/.

Henschel, P. (1999). Integration of play, learning and experience: What
museums afford the young. *Early Childhood Journal, 6*(3), 1–25.

Jensen, K. (2007). Routine HIV-testing policies. Bulletin of the World Health
Organization [online] 85(5). http://www.scielosp.org/scielo.php?
script=sci_arttext&pid=S0042-96862007000500028&lng=en&nrm=iso.

Jorgensen, C.H. (2005). School and workplace as learning environments in
VET. *Journal of Workplace Learning, 16*(8), 455–465.

Khathide, A.G. (2003). Teaching and talking about our sexuality: A means of
combating HIV/AIDS. In M.W. Dube (Ed.), *HIV/AIDS and the curriculum:
Methods of integrating HIV/AIDS in theological programmes* (pp. 1–9). Geneva:
WCC Publications.

Ndebele, P., Mfuso-Bengo, J., & Masiye, F. (2008). HIV reduces the relevance
of the principle of individual medical confidentiality among the Bantu people of Southern Africa. *Theoretical Medicine and Bioethics, 29*(5), 331–340.

Ntseane, P.G. (2004). *Thinking about behavioural change: An activity to raise consciousness and stimulate new thinking.* [HIV/AIDS dialogue]. Department of
Adult Education: University of Botswana.

Ntseane, P.G. (2006). Western and indigenous African knowledge systems
affecting gender and HIV/AIDS prevention in Botswana. In S.B. Merriam,
B.C. Courtney, & R.M. Cervero (Eds.), *Global issues and adult education:
Perspectives from Latin America, Southern Africa, and the United States* (pp. 219–
230). San Francisco: Jossey-Bass.

6 Health Care Professionals Working with Aboriginals: Canadian Adult Education and Practice

MARLENE ATLEO

The shift by the Canadian nation state from an assimilationist educational and health policy agenda for Aboriginals to one that supports self-determination must be formally recognized and integrated into educational programming at all levels, including formal schooling and informal learning in the community. Consequently, health care professionals working with Aboriginal people need to consider the socio-historical reality of colonial relationships in health care to reduce the reproduction of oppressive relationships in teaching and learning processes. They need to shift from a paternalistic relationship with Aboriginal people to one of dialogue and co-scription consistent with the principles of adult education articulated by Freire (1970, p. 84): 'One cannot expect positive results from an educational or political action program which fails to respect the particular view of the world held by the people. Such a program constitutes cultural invasion, good intentions notwithstanding. The starting point for organizing the program content of education or political action must be the present, existential, concrete situation, reflecting the aspirations of the people.'

Relevance for Aboriginal people requires that the present, existential, concrete, and aspirational aspects of their current lives be understood. As an example of how health and education coincide and sometimes collide, I supply here a case study that will then be analysed for its relevance. I use this story in the way that Randall recommends in chapter 11 of this book, as a means of unearthing truth and creating meaning with readers.

The Rushing Rapids Community Health Representative Goes to University

Rosie Swiftwater checked her iPhone and set it on vibrate as she entered the classroom. Nursing 1650: Community Nursing was a disappointment. After 10 years of working as the local community health representative (CHR) (NIICHRO, 2010) at home, in the remote northern community of Rushing Rapids, she had been asked to earn her Licensed Practical Nurse (LPN) credential so that she could provide more services for the nursing program of her tribal council. The contract nurses who came to the community stayed for shorter and shorter periods so that there was a real need for reliable community members to be trained to take over the health career roles and administration of the health services being devolved from First Nations and Inuit Health Branch (FNIHB), (Health Canada, 2010) to the tribal councils. Over the years, her role had changed from supporting the visiting nurse to coordinating the health services in the community and member visits to specialists down south. She was expected to know it all, and now they wanted her to be 'credentialed' too. This nursing course was about some other system of health care that she did not recognize. There were a lot of technicalities, core competencies, and Essential Skills (Human Resource Canada, 2006) to nursing that students needed to memorize and develop essays about, based in research that was about people and places other than Rushing Rapids. They even demanded she tell them about cultural competencies required or about community practice (Aboriginal Nurses Association, 2009) but there seemed to be very little about 'caring.'

The phone vibrated. Sheila Drinkwater, her relief CHR, was calling to tell her that Old Sally needed her diabetic ulcers taken care of, and to ask: Who was she to call about sending her out to the hospital? The professor's voice broke into her consciousness: 'Rosie, are you prepared to go first today?' First? Rosie tried to orient herself to the classroom. 'Sorry, Dr Whitelaw, I was fielding a call from my relief worker at home.' Whitelaw looked at her, 'You will have to be more focused in your coursework and turn that phone off when you are in my classroom!' Rosie looked around and found the class staring at her as if she was 'goofing off.' Damn! This one week a month for training did not work for her. The courses were interesting but hardly very useful. Rosie had assumed that Whitelaw knew about the realities of the conditions in which Rosie worked with the federal health care system through First Nations and Inuit Health (FNIHB). The grand chief and council had decided that credentialed health care workers were needed so that the health care programming could be devolved as part of the self-governance agenda over the next 10 years, and funding was currently available. So here she was down south at the university. Rosie sighed and looked around at the young students in the class. They were mostly the same age as her youngest child. She felt out of time and place. The desk she sat in was too small for her and the little armrest that served as a desk to write on did not come down all the way.

Dr Whitelaw was talking about diabetes in the Aboriginal community: 'Rosie? What is your community doing to reduce the levels of obesity and diabetes that are much higher than the national average?' Rosie felt her hackles rise as she was singled out in this classroom in front of the mainly non-Aboriginal students in this class. She wanted to shoot back: There was good food and healthy living before colonization, before residential schools, before the inadequate Indian and Northern Affairs Canada (INAC) (2010) housing, before the booze, before the drugs, before, before before…but she bit her tongue. She said, 'The First Nations and Inuit Health Branch is funding educational programming for communities about food and nutrition as well as diabetes foot care. Some of the older people have to go to the city for amputations as the disease progresses. It is difficult for them because the water system and supply is inadequate for the community needs. Milk is very expensive because it comes up by air. The winter road just did not last long enough for all the supplies to get in.' In a stage whisper, one of the young classmates said: 'Indians! They don't do anything for themselves. They get everything given to them, even fly the old ones to the city for treatment.' Whitelaw, ignoring the comment, said: 'But what are COMMUNITY MEMBERS doing to help themselves?' Rosie looked at her dumbfounded and sat silent. Should she feed into their ignorance and be damned with the credential her community needed? Rosie took a deep breath, ' Well, if you understand the treaty relationships, namely that we are all treaty people, you may begin to understand that Aboriginal health is not just an Aboriginal problem but a Canadian problem, created to a large extent by colonial policy and mindset of a settler society that projected European world views on indigenous North Americans.' Now the class and the professor were dumbfounded! She felt okay. It was a good start.

This case provides a clear example of the issues that arise in credentialing Aboriginals, and especially in mandating higher education. It raises questions about the meaning of shifts in public policy for professional education programs for Aboriginal people. It also raises questions about the challenges for Aboriginal students concerning university programming. These include issues related to academic, world view, and instructor knowledge of Aboriginal history and culture. For non-Aboriginal health educators, the history of Aboriginal/state relations is central to understanding the decolonizing process in which their practice is situated and how it is formally devolving in Canada. For Aboriginal health educators, the experience of health services is systematized and formalized to permit formal analysis. We need to ask about the challenges for non-Aboriginal health educators as well as for Aboriginal health educators. Finally, we wonder what kind of framework could be constructed so that there could be a meaningful dialogue between health care perspectives and philosophies and Aboriginal perspectives and philosophies.

How can health care professionals who have been immersed in a colonial history of indigenous exclusion and assimilation experience a transformation of practice that includes and celebrates Aboriginal people? Developing a discourse of cultural competency and proficiency in the context of anti-racist education (Nova Scotia, 2005) is probably the most important ongoing project in which Canada is currently engaged. Although Canada is theoretically a post-colonial settler nation, it continues on one hand to recruit increasing numbers of immigrants annually (Statistics Canada, 2006), and on the other hand continues to struggle in its relationships with its First People. The Aboriginal youth population is the fastest growing in the country, concentrated, according to Statistics Canada, in some centres, and population mobility is consonant with international and globalization trends. Canada, suggests Saul (2008), is challenged with fostering a coherent discourse of a nation state in which there is justice, room, and economic opportunity for all just inside the gateway of 'Essential Skills' (HRD, 2006). Professional and lay people participating in the co-construction of the discourse to provide equality of opportunity and outcomes are part of the legacy of adult education in Canada, and it is clear their work is ongoing (Welton, 2005). The nature of Canadian settler society in the context of Aboriginal homelands and colonial history is a challenging setting for this work, given the ways in which climate, geography, distances, geology, Canadian literature, the National Film Board, and the Canadian Broadcasting Corporation (CBC) have been shaped to mythologize the Canadian character and Aboriginal people therein. The insatiable national demand for population as human capital 'fuel' to meet the needs of nationhood continues a reli ance on a strategy of settlement or immigration, both as social reproduction and economic engines of settlement economies. How do health professions participate with burgeoning Aboriginal populations to meet their rights for recognition, respect, and justice based on Aboriginal rights recognized in the Canadian Constitution Act of 1982?

Colonial History: Evolution/Devolution/Revolution

Aboriginal health care as a project is the heart of my practice/praxis, the philosophy of my flesh; it is both academic and embodied. As a non-Aboriginal teenager who married into a remote First Nations community, my experience with health care provision for Aboriginals is filtered through 40-plus years of care. I wish that I could say it was filtered through my white privilege (Macintosh, 1988), but alas it was filtered through my status card[1] and the bodies of my husband, children, relatives, and friends. The colonized nature of the Aboriginal body is collateral damage of a colonial enterprise that obliterated coherent cultural systems of indigenous knowledge for wellness and health, erased them as superstitious nonsense over hundreds of years in Canada (Culhane Speck, 1987; Episkenew, 2009; Herring, Waldram, & Young, 2006; Kelm, 1998; Young, 1994). The subjective cultured body of the Cree, Nuu-chah-nulth, Anishnabe, Tlingit, Nisga, or Dene was replaced with a technical, de-cultured objectified body, birthed as a number under the Indian Act and in the dorms and hallways of the residential schools (Miller, 1997; Milloy, 1999).

On a personal level, as a status Indian under the 1951 amendment of the Indian Act,[2] my experience with 'Indian health' has been deeply humiliating, painful, and wrought with anxiety in its 'normlessness' and continuous change of system of bureaucracy culturally distanced from its clients. Those experiences were a major factor in my choice of occupational practice as an adult educator. First, I engaged in Aboriginal health promotion and then in the First Nations' Health Careers Program. What followed was a succession of health-related initiatives such as health and family science research, evaluation of health programs and projects, participatory action research, the development of an integrated community social and health organization. Latterly, my focus has been on the development, support, and ethics of health education and research in post-secondary institutions (Network Environments for Aboriginal Research in British Columbia (NEARBC)) (Atleo, 1997, 2008b). Aboriginal health as a field of study and practice was a means for me to articulate and mediate some of the service gaps I recognized in my community and beyond, which have been borne out by research over the last 40 years. I saw the role of education in preparing health professionals to work in cross-cultural situations, as well as its role in community development and political organization for systemic change.

My witness to the changes began in 1969 when I attended the graduation of my husband's aunt from a cohort program for community health representatives (CHRs) with Indian Health Training in Sardis, British Columbia. The CHRs, modelled after the barefoot doctors of China (Atleo, 2008a), were liaisons between their communities of origin and the health care practitioners from Medical Services,[3] which provides direct service to the communities. 'Indian Control of Indian Education' (National Indian Brotherhood, 1972) was the demand of indigenous people awakening to their own social, political, and moral legitimacies. Over the ensuing decades, I experienced the move from the devolution of programs and services of Indian Affairs and Health Canada to the evolution of programs and services by tribal councils, band governments, and extra tribal provincial and federal organizations. This devolution brought with it shifts in coverage of dental and medical benefits, bands and tribal councils taking over CHR positions, nursing programs devolving from Health Canada to Tribal Council jurisdiction, Non-Insured Health Benefits being managed at the tribal council level, and so on. This federally decentralizing evolution of the local health systems for First Nations, Métis, and Inuit Canadians creates a separate, distinct, and different reality, not tied to particular provinces or regions but integrated with the mainstream population and with the professionals serving Aboriginal populations.

The Zone of Aboriginal Education:
An Adult Learning Framework

My experience of moving across differing world views in both private and public life began to crystallize in my work on the social role attitudes of First Nations' mothers who juggle their dual cultural roles in the context of family life and occupational development (Atleo, 1993). Understanding the Zone of Aboriginal Education is recognizing that there are minimally two world views to which Aboriginal people are required to orient themselves: the academic official Canadian version and that of their experience and cultural community. As Freire (1970) stated above, for relevance the learners' reality must first be recognized. For example, Aboriginal mothers were expected to meet both local cultural standards for childrearing and formalized state childrearing standards simultaneously when the province took over welfare in the 1950s. The resultant 1960s' Scoop was a result of social workers not being able to acknowledge the multiple realities in which Aboriginal women were mothering. The internalized bicultural dialectic of movement between world views was, and remains, a challenge. In the Black American and African context it has been characterized as double consciousness, in which an inordinate amount of time is spent working to reconcile the two possibly antagonistic identities or orientations (Black, 2007). Double consciousness requires an educational strategy to expose its falseness. However, to be able to expose the falseness, the socio-historical construction of the lifeworld (Welton, 1995) and the levels of analysis of lifeworlds (Atleo, 2001) must be understood. Strategic adult education then requires instructors to understand this process and its implications as Aboriginal students deal with multiple orientations in their learning and literacy. Dialogic approaches to learning become important adult educational strategies to deal with such issues before specific instructional processes can be identified. What also must be understood is the manner in which such mystification colonizes the mind and hearts of people through use in education, and it becomes a requirement for educationalists that seek to promote equities through education to expose such practices (Atleo, 2008d).

Health Care Education for Health Care Professions

The challenge of changing teaching strategies and styles across world views needs to be acknowledged at the onset (Aboriginal Nurses Association, 2009). The work on cross-cultural research (Lonner & Berry, 1986) and psychological development (Kim & Berry, 1993) has largely been absent from the educationalist literature. More recently the discourse has been about colonization and decolonization in the spirit of Smith's work (1999). But it would seem that it is not an either/or issue, in particular in the health sciences world where the elitist and Eurocentric legacy of the scientific mindset comes sharply into focus. Aboriginal ways of being and knowing can clash with scientific ways of being and knowing if there is insufficient brokering of curriculum and instruction on the two ways of thinking about and being in the world. For non-Aboriginal instructors and institutions to develop capacity and confer legitimacy to indigenous ways of knowing and teaching requires that their teaching approaches be accounted for and their efficacy demonstrable in indigenous ways of knowing and being. How else can the educational systems/institutions certify the courses or programming for particular populations? The development of a research program that maps the terrain of Aboriginal peoples from an emic (insider) perspective has been a recent development (McNaughton & Rock, 2003). In this kind of research, there arise the issues of ethical interaction with individuals from different world views (Piquemal, 2004) – in particular, as it is related to the field practice of the researchers and the clinical aspects of practice that are necessary to achieve competency in the techno-rational aspects of coursework, preceptorships, and field adaptations (Aboriginal Nurses Association, 2009). Then there is the issue of moral equality between individuals while teaching, given that some teachers may not be proficient and even ignorant of such basics as cultural ways of being and knowing, child care, and everyday life (Atleo, 1990 1993; Keitlah, 1995). It becomes obvious that teaching across lifeworlds (Welton, 1995), the sum total of our existence, creates problems of structure and function, power, and legitimacy. Then there is the question of which content fits into which context from whose point of view, and the risk of misunderstanding and continued oppression increases.

Mediating the lifeworld in relationships and education is a challenge that requires educators to understand both teacher and learner and the cultures in which they are embedded. So it should not be surprising that from early encounters with colonizers, Aboriginal peoples identified the parallel structure between their cognitive mindsets and lifeworlds and those of the newcomers. The articulation of this in metaphor is the two-row wampum belt (Bonaparte, 2005), and in analogous or relational reasoning articulated by of the ways and means with which to negotiate relationships and attention across cultures. A recent example of a metaphor developed through focus group methodology can be found in the interactive learning models of First Nations, Inuit, and Métis learning (Canadian Council of Learning, 2009). The two-row wampum model suggests the power relations were relatively equal, whereas in the CCL models the close relationship is invisible. Shifting power relations over time suggest that there are also learning responses to different ways of making meaning between world views (from assimilation to accommodation to dialogue). To move between world views, even with metaphorical models, requires intimate knowledge of and experience in both world views, because it is a subjective rather than an objective journey.

The medicine wheel models, articulated as Aboriginal methodology that proliferate in the Aboriginal health literature, can be understood as a project to incorporate Western ideas into circle thinking (e.g.,

Graveline; 2000; McCormick & Wong, 2006), and to present them as indigenous cultural models reflecting Aboriginal ways of thinking. Once textualized and embedded in curriculum, the medicine wheel becomes a powerful concept map in which to assimilate ideas. While such models may represent some indigenous world views, they are not necessarily generalizable to all Aboriginal populations. The medicine wheel is thus reminiscent of the hermeneutic circle (Geanellos, 2003), which is familiar to nursing practice and research, and may well seem to be a satisfactory conceptual tool. However, Geanellos (2003) cautions that the use of this method of inquiry carries with it an obligation to acknowledge the philosophical implications and contextual understandings of moving between two disparate world views grounded in different continents and histories. This includes presuppositions and assumptions, accuracy about meanings in translation, and outcomes that are part of all teaching encounters but may be particularly problematic across cultures. This would apply to circle research and teaching in which the hermeneutic logic must be worked through levels of analysis in developing understanding of the situation or case study.

For Aboriginal health education this would require both the instrumental knowledge of the nursing curriculum (e.g., protocols, anatomical facts, math to calculate dosages) as well as relational brokering of the same by an instructor well versed in cross-cultural practice (e.g., how to address students, how to interact, how to support their aspirations). Adult learners, including Aboriginal learners, require relevance to maintain motivation (Kirkness & Barnhardt, 1991). This is completely consistent with the tenets of adult learning and education. How can educators make the material RELEVANT to students? Educators need to ask themselves: What are the salient critical dis-ease issues in Aboriginal communities for Aboriginal people (Reading, 2009)? How do Indigenous people see their decolonization (Smith, 1999) through health services and methodologies? What happens when Aboriginal people challenge the status quo of the medical models developed in the context of colonial states (Tait, 2003) in which the victim is blamed for the context of colonization (e.g., fetal alcohol syndrome)? Do we continue with pathologizing practices (Shields, Bishop, & Mazawi, 2004), or do we as adult educators enter a new hermeneutic circle that recognizes the multiplicity of indigenous ways of being and knowing (Tully, 1995) and begin a true dialogue (Shields & Edwards, 2005) with Aboriginal students? As teachers and facilitators, do we meet learners in their own world view as self-knowing practitioners or do we require them to move into our ways of being and knowing? Do we understand our own situated-ness, the pretexts and presuppositions of the profession with which we enter into the learning circle, where we speak as moral and social equals (Fitznor, 2002)?

To begin to deal with some of these multiplicities, three professional bodies worked together to develop a framework in which to craft a common discourse in health care (Aboriginal Nurses Association of Canada, 2009). The ANAOC, together with the Canadian Nurses Association (CNA) and the Canadian Association of Schools of Nursing (CASN), identified several core competencies for nursing practice with Aboriginal people: (a) post-colonial understanding, (b) intercultural communication strategies, (c) inclusivity, (d) respect, (e) indigenous knowledge, and (f) mentoring and support of students for success. These core competencies are based in a view of professional competency in primary health care delivery. These competencies are further elaborated through the recognition of principles that include the recognition of culture with an analysis of principles and assumptions of culture. The manner in which power and privilege operate in different cultures, how difference is expressed and resources are distributed, as well as how racism and oppression are encountered in health care contexts, are central themes in this framework. Anti-racist and cultural competency and proficiency strategies and education must be the basis for the development of adult education teaching and learning in Aboriginal health because both Aboriginal and non-Aboriginal people are involved in unequal relationships. Both Aboriginals and non-Aboriginals must become mutually self-conscious en route to mutual participation in health and healing of Canadians of Aboriginal ancestry.

In the Canadian health care system we may have Aboriginal people cared for by non-Aboriginal health care professionals or taught by them in professional practice. However, we may also have Aboriginal people care for and teach non-Aboriginal people. Thus the topic of Aboriginal health care education is rife with issues of positionality and position taking. Cross-cultural methodologies (Denzin, Lincoln, & Smith, 2008; Kim & Berry, 1993; Lonner & Berry, 1986; Smith, 1999) based in emic (or community insider) perspectives and ethos have found that there is a preference for 'healing' and 'wellness' as concepts to describe the states of embodiment being desired. In contrast, etic (outsider) perspectives prefer the term 'health,' which accrues to the more techno-rational and science-based ways of discussing Aboriginal bodies and bodies in general (emic/etic) (Lonner & Berry, 1986). Membership in communities of practice comes with literary power (Janks, 2010) that requires health practitioners to recognize the embodiments of social developmental trajectories that have their own knowledge and practice and ways of being. For Canadian Aboriginal people, this distinctness is still reflected in the two-row wampum, which is alive and well in Canadian Aboriginal discourse after 350 years. It is time to bring it into the foreground to employ as a foundation to dialogically co-construct a new way of being with each other in the Canadian health care context.

Beyond the Wampum Belt Model of Indigenous and Settler Relations

While indigenous people, families, and communities have been the focus of assimilationist laws and policies for centuries, in 1982 the Canadian Constitution recognized Aboriginal people as indigenous to the territory of the Canadian nation state and recognized their undefined Aboriginal rights. In 1988, the Canadian federal government acknowledged the enduring group identities of ethnic individuals by legally assuring multiculturalism. This ensured the unique human capital of ethnic minorities in their selective interaction with Canadian social and economic institutions. Multiculturalism legally changed the relationship between immigrant and Aboriginal social norms and the norms of the larger society from one of exclusion (dominant cultural expression valued) to one of inclusion in which pluralistic cultural expressions are valued (Atleo, 1990). This fundamental change from an exclusive to an inclusive orientation requires profound changes in the orientations of education and health professionals throughout the governance systems, from policy administration to field adjustments in specific practice. Such changes require health and adult education specialists to investigate changes in value expressions, as well as the social impact of shifts at a policy level, and the need for re-education of health professionals. Recognition and respect for the personhood of the learner requires that expert professionals broker the cultural knowledge to the learner using adult education strategies.

Writing in 1997, I asked whether the development of a discourse of First Nations healing was a means of providing better health using objective measures for First Nations people through changes in the health care delivery systems, or if it was another means of domination of First Nations, since it required them to adapt to the needs of the Euroheritage system (Atleo, 1997). While the jury is still out on that question, this last decade has seen the beginning of Canadian health care systems, professionals, professional organizations, and education systems to systematically address Aboriginal needs and aspirations through an increasingly equitable discourse. Such change comes in the context of international pressure to recognize indigenous rights; with legal requirements to consult Aboriginal people about resource extraction where Aboriginal land rights remain. Such change comes with the rising health care costs originating from the burden of exclusion and poverty on the physical bodies of increasing numbers of Aboriginal people across Canada. Such change comes in the face of a growing Aboriginal youth population with a need for education to ameliorate such conditions in order to reduce further alienation of Aboriginal people in a culturally fragmented nation state. In the academy, change has been creeping in for 40 years, with courses and programs of study and faculties of Native Studies, First Nations, Aboriginal, and Indigenous Studies. There are demands that Indigenous (IK) and/or Traditional Knowledge (TK) be either integrated throughout programming or minimally instituted through stand alone courses to meet local demands for student enrolment and retention (M. Atleo, 2006; R. Atleo, 1999a, 1999b). And, finally, such change comes based on the sheer demand for home-grown Canadian human resources that are not readily recruited or maintained via immigration. Under these conditions of change, Aboriginal people are again in a position to become allies of the Canadian state based in history and in indigenous knowledge of the territory called Canada that stretches from sea to sea to sea. Adult health care education can be central to such a project for the good of all in the work of 'the reconciliation of the pre-existence of Aboriginal societies with the sovereignty of the Crown. Let us face it, we are all here to stay' (Chief Justice H.A. Hutcheon, Government of British Columbia, 1997), since as adult educators 'we make the road by walking' (Bell, Gaventa, & Peters, 1991).

NOTES

1 The Indian Status Card is a piece of identification issued by agents authorized by Indian Affairs to certify those individuals who have legal status under the Indian Act. The Indian Act: http://www.bloorstreet.com/sindact.htm#4.

2 The 1951 amendment of the Indian Act legislated that non-Indian females who married status Indian males became de facto status Indians, as did their offspring and any minor children they may have had from previous relationships.

3 Medical Services was the Indian Health division of Health Canada. Currently, First Nations and Inuit Health fill that function.

REFERENCES

Aboriginal Nurses Association of Canada. (2009). Cultural competence and cultural safety in nursing education: A framework for First Nations, Inuit and Métis nursing. Retrieved 1 September 2011 from http://www.anac.on.ca/Documents/Making%20It%20Happen%20Curriculum%20Project/FINALFRAMEWORK.pdf.

Atleo, M. (1990). Studying Canadian indigenous families: A special case of ethnicity in a multicultural nation. In Jeanne M. Hilton (Ed.), Papers of the Western Region Home Management and Family Economics Educators (pp. 35–43). Reno, NV: Department of Human Resources and Family Studies, University of Nevada.

Atleo, M. (1993). Social role attitudes and the planning behaviour of First Nations mothers with school age children. Unpublished MA thesis. Vancouver: University of British Columbia.

Atleo, M. (1997). First Nations healing: Dominance or health? The Canadian Journal for the Study of Adult Education, 11(2), 63–77.

Atleo, M. (2006, 27–31 May). First Nations program development in post secondary settings: Malaspina University College and other models. Aboriginal education: Issues in leadership. Toronto: Canadian Association of Studies in Educational Administration, CSSE, York University.

Atleo, M. (2008a). Decolonizing Canadian Aboriginal health and social services from the inside out: A case study – The Ahousaht Holistic Society. In Kerstin Knopf (Series Ed.), Aboriginal peoples in Canada in the 21st Century (pp. 42–61). Ottawa: University of Ottawa Press.

Atleo, M. (2008b, 14 February). From policy to praxis and back again: Are there 'rules' of knowledge translation across bodies/world views? Network Environments for Aboriginal Research in British Columbia: NEARBC. Victoria, BC: University of Victoria: Aboriginal Health Research Network. Retrieved 10 October 2011 from http://www.nearbc.ca/documents/2008/M-Atleo.pdf.

Atleo, M. (2008c). Indigenous learning models in the context of socio-economic change: A storywork approach. In Wesley Heber (Series Ed.), Indigenous education: Asia/Pacific (pp. 21–32). Regina, SK: Indigenous Studies Research Centre, First Nations University.

Atleo, M.R. (2008d). Strategies for equities in indigenous education: A Canadian First Nations case study. In Adolfo de Oliveira (Ed.), Routledge studies in anthropology: Decolonizing indigenous rights (pp. 132–164). London: Routledge.

Atleo, M.R. (1999a). Guest editorial: A long term perspective of First Nations educational experience. The Learning Quarterly (Special issue, First Nations Studies: The Malaspina Success), 3(1), 2–5. http://www.eric. ed.gov/PDFS/ED450840.pdf.

Atleo, M.R. (1999b). First Nations studies at Malaspina University College: The vision. The Learning Quarterly [Special issue, First Nations Studies: The Malaspina Success], 3(1), 6–11. http://www.eric.ed.gov/PDFS/ ED450840.pdf.

Atleo, M.R., & James, A. (2000). Oral tradition – A literacy for lifelong learning: Native American approaches to justice and wellness education. In T.J. Sork, V-L. Chapman, & R. St. Clair (Eds.). Proceedings of the 41st Annual Adult Education Research Conference, 2–4 June 2000 (pp. 535–536). Vancouver: University of British Columbia. Retrieved 22 November 2009 from http://www.eric.ed.gov/ERICDocs/data/ericdocs2sql/content_ storage_01/0000019b/80/16/fd/a1.pdf.Bell, B., Gaventa, J., & Peters, J. (Eds.). (1991). We make the road by walking: Conversations on education and social change: Myles Horton & Paulo Freire. Philadelphia: Temple University Press.

Black, M. (2007). Fanon and DuBoisian double consciousness. Human Architecture: Journal of the Sociology of Self-Knowledge, 5 (Special issue), 393–404.

Bonaparte, D. (2005). The two row wampum belt: An Akwesasne tradition of vessel and canoe. Retrieved 10 October 2011 from http://www.wampum chronicles.com/tworowwampumbelt.html.

Canadian Council of Learning. (2009). The state of Aboriginal learning in Canada: A holistic approach to measuring success. Retrieved 10 October 2011 from http://www.ccl-cca.ca/CCL/Reports/StateofAboriginalLearning? Language=EN.

Culhane Speck, D. (1987). An error in judgment: The politics of medical care in an Indian / white community. Vancouver: Talonbooks.

Denzin, N.K., Lincoln, Y.S., & Smith, L.T. (Eds.). (2008). Handbook of critical and indigenous methodologies. Thousand Oaks, CA: Sage.

Episkenew, J. (2009). Taking back our spirits: Indigenous literature, public policy, and healing. Winnipeg: University of Manitoba Press.

Fitznor, L. (2002). Aboriginal educators' stories: Rekindling Aboriginal world views. PhD thesis. OISE/University of Toronto.

Freire, P. (1970). Pedagogy of the oppressed. New York: Herder and Herder.

Geanellos, R. (2003). Hermeneutic philosophy. Part I: Implications of its use as methodology in interpretive nursing research. Nursing Inquiry, 5(3), 154–163.

Government of British Columbia. (1997). Delgamuukw v. British Columbia. File no. 23799, 1997: 16, 17 June; 1997: 11 December. Paragraph 186.

Graveline, F.J. (2000). Circle as methodology: Enacting an Aboriginal paradigm. International Journal for Qualitative Studies in Education, 13(4), 361–370.

Health Canada. (2010). First Nations, Inuit and Aboriginal health branch. Retrieved 1 October 2011 from http://www.hc-sc.gc.ca/fniah-spnia/pubs/promotion/_2009-2010/index-eng.php.

Herring, A., Waldram, J., & Young K.T. (2006). Aboriginal health in Canada: Historical, cultural, and epidemiological perspectives. Toronto: University of Toronto Press.

Human Resource Canada. (2006). Essential skills. Retrieved 10 October 2011 from http://www.hrsdc.gc.ca/eng/workplaceskills/essential_skills/general/home.shtml.

Indian and Northern Affairs Canada. (2010). About INAC. Retrieved 1 January 2010 from http://www.ainc-inac.gc.ca/ai/index-eng.asp.

Janks, H. (2010). Literacy and power. In Sonia Nieto (Series Editor), Language, Culture, and Teaching. New York: Routledge.

Keitlah, W. (1995). Wawaaciakuk yaqwii?itquu?as: The sayings of our first people. Penticton, BC: Theytus Books.

Kelm, M.E. (1998). Colonizing bodies: Aboriginal health and healing in British Columbia, 1900–50. Vancouver: University of British Columbia Press.

Kirkness, V.J., & Barnhardt, R. (1991). First Nations and higher education: The four R's – respect, relevance, reciprocity, responsibility. Journal of American Indian Education, 30(3), 1–15.

Kim, U., & Berry, J.W. (Eds.). (1993). Indigenous psychologies: Research and experience in cultural context. Cross-cultural research and methodology series. Vol.8. Newbury Park, CA: Sage.

Lonner, W.J., & Berry, J.W. (Eds.). (1986). Field methods in cross-cultural research. Cross-cultural research and methodology series. Vol. 8. Beverly Hills, CA: Sage.

McCormick, R., & Wong, P.T.P. (2006). Coping and resilience in Aboriginal people. In P.T.P. Wong & L.C.J. Wong (Eds.), Handbook of multicultural perspectives on stress and coping (pp. 515–533). New York: Springer.

McIntosh, P. (1988). White privilege and male privilege: A personal account of coming to see correspondences in women's studies. Center for Research on Women, Wellesley College, MA 02181. Retrieved 22 November 2010 from http://www.iub.edu/~tchsotl/part2/McIntosh%20White%20Privilege.pdf.

McNaughton, C., & Rock, D. (2003). Opportunities in Aboriginal research results of SSHRC's dialogue on research and Aboriginal peoples. Ottawa: Social

Sciences and Humanities Research Council. Retrieved 10 January 2011 from http://www.sshrc-crsh.gc.ca/funding-financement/apply-demande/background-renseignements/aboriginal_backgrounder_e.pdf.

Miller, J.M. (1997). Shingwaulk's vision: A history of Native residential schools. Toronto: University of Toronto Press.

Milloy, J. (1999). A national crime: The Canadian government and the residential school system – 1879 to 1986. Winnipeg: University of Manitoba Press.

National Indian Brotherhood. (1972). Indian control of Indian education. Ottawa: National Indian Brotherhood.

National Indian and Inuit Community Health Representatives Organization. (2010). Aboriginal human health resources. Retrieved 10 October 2011 from http://www.niichro.com/2004/?page=reports&lang=en.

Nova Scotia. (2005). A cultural competence guide for primary health care professionals in Nova Scotia. Retrieved 10 October 2011 from http://www.healthteamnovascotia.ca/cultural_competence/Cultural_Competence_guide_for_Primary_Health_Care_Professionals.pdf.

Piquemal, N. (2004). Relational ethics in cross-cultural teaching: Teacher as researcher Canadian Journal of Educational Administration and Policy. Issue #32. Retrieved 10 October 2011 from http://www.umanitoba.ca/publications/cjeap/articles/noma/relationalethics.piquemal.html.

Reading, J. (2009). The crisis of chronic disease among Aboriginal peoples: A challenge for public health, population health and social policy. Victoria, BC: Centre for Aboriginal Health, University of Victoria.

Saul, J.R. (2008). A fair country: Telling truths about Canada. Toronto: Penguin Press.

Shields, C.M., & Edwards, M.M. (2005). Dialogue is not just talk: A new ground for educational leadership. New York: Peter Lang.

Shields, C.M., Bishop, R., & Mazawi, A.E. (2004). Pathologizing practices: The impact of deficit thinking on education. Counterpoints Series: Studies in postmodern theory of education. New York: Peter Lang.

Smith, L.T. (1999). Decolonizing methodologies: Research and indigenous peoples. London: Zed.

Statistics Canada. (2006). Aboriginal peoples: 2006 census. Retrieved 10 October 2011 from http://www.statcan.gc.ca/bsolc/olc-cel/olc-cel?lang=eng&catno=97-558-X.

Tait, C. (2003). The tip of the iceberg: The making of fetal alcohol syndrome in Canada. Unpublished PhD dissertation, McGill University, Montreal.

Tully, J. (1995). Strange multiplicities: Constitutionalism in an age of diversity. Cambridge: Cambridge University Press.

Welton, M.R. (1995). In defense of the lifeworld: Critical perspectives on adult learning. New York: SUNY Press.

Welton, M.R. (2005). Designing the just learning society: A critical inquiry. Cardiff, UK: National Institute of Adult Continuing Education.

Young, K.T. (1994). The health of Native Americans: Towards a bio-cultural epidemiology. London: Oxford University Press.

7 Literacy and Health: Implications for Health and Education Professionals

BARBARA RONSON AND IRVING ROOTMAN

In the past few decades we have learned much about how many people are affected by low literacy skills, and how such skills are related to poorer health outcomes. Professionals working in both health and education can benefit by knowing the importance of this relationship and by becoming familiar with examples of how research in this field can be used to improve their practice.

There are many definitions of 'health,' 'literacy,' and the intermediating concept 'health literacy' – and there is no consensus yet. Perhaps most often, people think of health as the absence of disease. At least this is how it is frequently viewed in clinical contexts (e.g., Critchley, 1978, p. 784). Yet, health is defined more holistically in the constitution of the World Health Organization (WHO, 1946) as a 'state of complete physical, mental, and social well-being and not merely the absence of disease and infirmity' (p. 1).

Although one might think that the WHO definition would find international acceptance, it has, in fact, been repeatedly criticized, mostly because it puts no boundaries on what is possible to encompass by the term health (hence there is no limit on expenditure) (Rootman & Raeburn, 1994, p. 58). The WHO definition was elaborated in the 1986 Ottawa Charter for Health Promotion as 'a resource for everyday life, not the objective of living' (WHO, 1986), further drawing attention to a holistic understanding with broader determinants. This broader determinants perspective is reflected by many authors in this book, including English and Moseley. From the other end of the spectrum, the WHO definition has been criticized for not going beyond the concept of physical, mental, and social skills; for example, by including a 'spiritual' component. This issue was addressed at the 2005 WHO Conference on Health Promotion in Bangkok and is reflected in the Bangkok Charter for

Health Promotion, which suggested that health promotion also encompasses 'spiritual well-being' (WHO, 2005).

In the research literature, health is often estimated by indicators such as blood pressure, cholesterol level, or time missed from work or school. Other times, it is assessed by asking people to self-report. The health of groups or cohorts can be estimated by the levels of morbidity (the incidence of certain conditions such as diabetes, cancer, or obesity) and by mortality (the average age of death and incidence of death at different age levels). Spiritual, emotional, and mental health of groups has sometimes been estimated by the incidence of suicide, depression, and other psychiatric indicators.

The 1991 U.S. National Literacy Act defines literacy as 'an individual's ability to read, write and speak in English, and compute and solve problems at levels of proficiency necessary to function on the job and in society, to achieve one's goals, and develop one's knowledge and potential' (United States Congress, House Committee on Education and Labour, 1991, p. 2). Similarly, the Canadian Expert Panel on Health Literacy defines it as 'the ability to understand and use reading, writing, speaking and other forms of communication as ways to participate in society and achieve one's goals and potential' (Rootman & Gordon-El-Bihbety, 2008, p. 10).

Early measures of literacy were simple tests of whether one could read a short paragraph out loud, or sign one's name on a marriage certificate. In the past, literacy rates were estimated by years of education, a factor that shows higher correlation with health than socio-economic status, income, or occupation (Ronson & Rootman, 2009), but is not as precise. Daily reading activity, for example, probably has more of an impact on literacy levels than years of education (Canadian Council on Learning, 2008). More recently, literacy has been measured in large-scale national- and international surveys such as the *International Adult Literacy Survey* (Statistics Canada, 1994) and its successor, the *International Adult Literacy and Skills Survey* (Statistics Canada, 2003) in both of which Canada was an early participant. These surveys have measured people's abilities to read prose, do arithmetic computations, and use documents such as maps, graphs, and application forms in order to 'participate in society and achieve one's goals and potential' (Rootman & Gordon-El-Bihbety, p. 10). Based on the analysis of the 2003 IALSS for Canada, about 12 million adult Canadians were estimated to be below the minimum required level of proficiency in prose and document literacy (48%), though most of these people develop coping skills and hide the issue from others. The great majority of those classified as below the minimum required level were native speakers of English or French including many who graduated from Canadian secondary and post-secondary schools. For many practitioners in the health and other professions, this was shocking information.

Moreover, researchers have found a very high correlation between low reading skills and poor health in the last few decades. For example, lower literacy scores have been found to be related to longer hospitalizations (Baker, Parker, Williams, Clark, & Nurss, 1997; Baker et al., 2002); higher rates of cervical cancer (Lindau, Tamori, Lyons, Langseth, Bennett, & Garcia, 2002); poorer self-reported health (Canadian Council on Learning, 2007; Mossey & Shapiro, 1982); and mortality rates from 50 per cent higher (Baker, Wolf, Feinglass, Thompson, Guzmararian, & Huang, 2007) to 200 per cent higher (Sudore et al., 2006) among some populations, even after adjusting for numerous variables such as socio-economic status and health-related behaviours. According to one study, low reading proficiency is the second strongest predictor of mortality after smoking, and a more powerful variable than either income or years of education (Baker et al., 2007).

Because of the growing interest in the relationship between health and literacy, and the related area of multi-literacies, an intermediary construct, *health literacy*, is increasingly used, and is now considered something that could potentially be measured and that health promoters could be accountable for (Nutbeam, 2000). Health literacy was defined by the Canadian Expert Panel on Health Literacy as 'the ability to access, understand, evaluate and communicate information as a way to promote, maintain and improve health in a variety of settings across the life-course' (Rootman & Gordon-El-Bihbety, 2008, p. 11). In Europe and the United States, definitions are similar (Kickbusch, 2007; Zarcadoolas, Pleasant, & Greer, 2005, pp. 196–197). Though definitions vary, there is an increasing recognition that there are two sides to health literacy: the skills that individuals bring to health situations and the abilities of health professionals and institutions to provide health information effectively. According to the United States' Institute of Medicine Expert Committee on Health Literacy, an individual's capacity and skills are equally important as the health context, or 'range of environments and situations related to health' that they encounter (Nielsen-Bohlman, Panzer, & Kindig, 2004, p. 32). Health literacy arises from the interaction of the individual and the health context. Thus, the onus should not be on individuals alone to solve the problem by improving their skills. Health care practitioners and media also play an important role.

Furthermore, there appears to be significant differences between the relationships of literacy to health and health literacy to health. Specifically, general literacy, however defined, tends to be related to health in terms of its impact on larger determinants of health such as employment and income, which in turn have an impact on exposure to health risks and life circumstances in general and on health and quality of life (Rootman & Ronson, 2005). Health literacy, on the other hand, has a more direct impact on short-term health through health behaviours and decisions that people make about their health (Rootman & Ronson). Of particular concern is the ability of people to follow directions for taking prescription medicine, prepare baby formula, and understand nutritional content information on food packaging and safety information on the job. Errors in these matters result in multiple hospitalizations and even deaths in hospitals every day.

Figure 7.1, which follows, was developed by the authors with input from practitioners, to provide a comprehensive overview of the relationships among general literacy, health literacy, and other literacies, as well as their possible consequences and determinants.

Health literacy has been measured by a variety of tests (e.g., Newest Vital Sign (NVS); Rapid Estimate of Literacy and Medicine (REALM); Test of Functional Health Literacy in Adults (TOHFLA)). More recently, a subset of tasks related to health on national and international literacy studies have been used to assess and study broad levels of health literacy retroactively, and even larger numbers of Canadians have been found to be below the required level on health literacy than on literacy. This is likely because health literacy requires skills in addition to literacy, such as those needed to find health information, evaluate it and integrate it from a variety of sources, as well as some special knowledge such as the vocabulary of health and the culture of the health system. In 2003, an estimated 11.7 million working-age residents of Canada (55%) appeared to lack the minimum level of health literacy needed to effectively manage their health information needs (Canadian Council on Learning, 2007). When seniors are added, an estimated 14.8 million were lacking adequate health literacy skills; which includes almost 90 per cent of people over the age of 65. If these estimates are accurate, there are large numbers of adults in Canada who do not have adequate skills in English or French to manage their health. Health care practitioners and educators need to take this into account as they will undoubtedly encounter many of them in their work and need to be adequately prepared.

Figure 7.1. General, Health, and Other Literacies

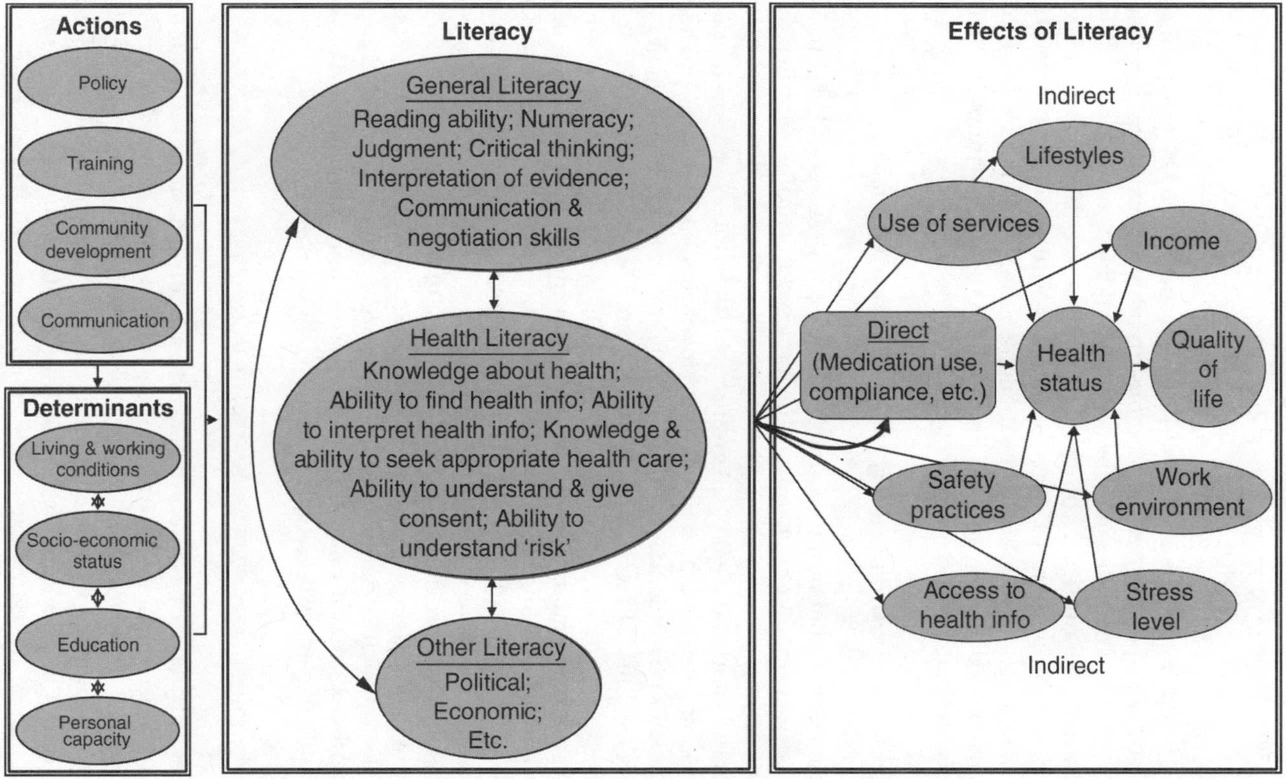

Actions
- Policy
- Training
- Community development
- Communication

Determinants
- Living & working conditions
- Socio-economic status
- Education
- Personal capacity

Literacy

General Literacy
Reading ability; Numeracy; Judgment; Critical thinking; Interpretation of evidence; Communication & negotiation skills

Health Literacy
Knowledge about health; Ability to find health info; Ability to interpret health info; Knowledge & ability to seek appropriate health care; Ability to understand & give consent; Ability to understand 'risk'

Other Literacy
Political; Economic; Etc.

Effects of Literacy

Indirect
- Lifestyles
- Income
- Quality of life
- Use of services
- Health status
- Work environment
- Stress level
- Safety practices
- Access to health info

Direct (Medication use, compliance, etc.)

Indirect

Interventions

Research in literacy and health has led health practitioners to reach out to health educators and adult learners, and vice versa. Such collaborations can open up new possibilities for adult educators and health care providers. The following types of collaborative interventions will be discussed: (a) improving comprehensibility of health education materials; (b) combining plain language materials with training; (c) developing curricula for health literacy; (d) empowering learners to be health advisors and educators; and (e) developing ongoing partnerships between health agencies and educational institutions.

Improving Comprehensibility of Health Education Materials

One of the common ways that health care professionals have drawn on the field of adult education is through an effort to present health care information to patients and consumers in a form that can be readily understood and used by all groups, including those with low literacy levels. Many studies have shown that much health literature provided to patients is written at a reading level higher than the average patient possesses (Rudd, Epstein Anderson, Oppenheimer, & Nath, 2007; Nielsen-Bohlman, Panzer, & Kindig, 2004). This has led to a serious effort to measure readability levels of health education materials and reading ability of consumers, and to use plain language and audiovisual tools to increase the effectiveness of non-verbal, supplementary health information for patients. In many cases, adult literacy students have assisted health care providers develop or translate health education material into *plain language* (Lawrence & Soricone, 2005; Petch, Levitt, & Levitt, 2004), which is defined as 'a way of organizing and presenting information so that it's easy for people to read and understand' (Canadian Public Health Association, n.d.).

Combining Plain Language Materials with Training

Several studies have shown that when plain language health information is accompanied by training, greater benefits are possible (Clement, Ibrahim, Crichton, Wolf, & Rowlands, 2009). For example, a United States study led by Ariella Herman of the UCLA/Johnson and Johnson Health Care Institute, found that training Head Start families on the use of an easy-to-read resource in English or Spanish had a positive impact both on the health of families and on health care costs (Institute for Healthcare Advancement, 2009). Gains were made not only in comparison to a demographically matched control group, but also in comparison to families who received the plain language resource without training. Early results showed that parents became more knowledgeable about what to do when their children got sick, and when to go to a clinic or emergency department. The cost savings to Medicare were calculated to be about $550 per family for a program that cost about $60 per family, or about 5 million annually for every 10,000 families served (UCLA press release, November 2007). As well, participant families reported considerably fewer absences from work and school after training with the program. The project has been refined and expanded across the United States with about 14,000 families participating to date.

Developing Curricula for Health Literacy

Several efforts have been made to develop curricula on health tailored to adult literacy classes (Corrigan, Bodane, & Rischbieter, 1994; Levy et al., 2008; McMillan, 2007; Rudd & Comings, 1994). One of the most extensive recent efforts to develop and pilot test a health curriculum for adults with low literacy levels, Skilled for Health (SfH) has taken place in England with support from the Department of Health and other organizations (ContinYou, 2010). Between 2003 and 2006 community-based learning materials were produced on multiple health topics, and from 2007 to 2009 they were pilot tested in 17 centres across the United Kingdom. The idea was to attract people who would not ordinarily sign up for adult education classes using health as a hook. Life and literacy skills were embedded into health topics, and it was hoped that participants might sign up for further upgrading of skills for lifelong learning. Participants could select which health topics they wished to study. Preliminary evaluation results suggested that the materials were well received (with an 80% retention rate) and freely adapted for local use, complemented in some cases by exercise programs and other components. Health was a significant incentive to join for some participants, while learning English was another, especially for those with other mother tongues. Participants' health knowledge increased significantly after taking the SfH curriculum, particularly in the areas of healthy eating, exercising, smoking, drinking, and mental health. Behavioural changes such as increased fruit and vegetable consumption and exercise were also noted. The program created motivation to continue learning, with 25 per cent registering for further courses. It also raised language skill levels of some participants.

Though we have come a long way in improving the quality of health curricula for learners over the years, it is still often erroneously assumed that measurable literacy or health literacy levels can be easily improved among adults, even with teachers from other disciplines. However, a study by Levy and others (2008) from the University of Illinois showed that a 42-hour curriculum on health literacy piloted in 42 adult literacy centres across the state, involving over 2000 adult basic education (ABE) and English for speakers of other languages (ESOL) students, did not change literacy levels, though clear health knowledge gains were observed for students at all levels of literacy, compared to no gains among control students.

Empowering Learners to be Health Advisors and Educators

Empowerment, a key concept of the Ottawa Charter for Health Promotion (WHO, 1986), has increasingly been adopted as a principle of health education and improvement projects. Accordingly, an effort has been made to give more decision-making power and opportunities to consumers and learners. In the early 1990s Norton and Horne (1998) worked with 14 women in a literacy class in Edmonton to develop health programs on topics of their choice. Programs included units on stress, saying no, anger, diet and exercise, menopause, and living healthily on a low budget. Together, they developed programs which were field tested at four sites in the two years that followed. Learners reported some improvements in their own health practices, including lowering fat and sodium in their diets and managing stress and anger better, as a result of their participation in this supportive, creative group.

At about the same time, Marcia Hohn (1998) piloted an 'empowerment model' for training learners as health curriculum developers and advisors in Massachusetts. She followed key principles of participation, empowerment, democracy, and power-sharing – ideas that have some footing in a number of fields including health promotion. Together, Hohn and her student 'Health Action Team' chose two topics to prepare to teach: early detection of certain cancers, and family violence. For each area, they developed three-part programs of five hours, which were delivered in six different classrooms over a period of four months, reaching over 150 students. Their work led to the development of a four-part teaching and learning process that can be applied to any health issue: (a) providing basic information, (b) hands-on activities for teaching skills and tools, (c) drama to bring out difficult issues for discussion, and (d) providing and discussing resources for the next steps or for obtaining further assistance.

Hohn (1998) concluded that empowerment health education enhances the potential for sustained individual and collective action about health. Furthermore, adult literacy programs, including English language, family literacy, general educational development, and basic literacy programs provide ideal sites for reaching out to low literacy communities that have been disconnected from traditional health education and promotion efforts. The qualitative data she presents in her study show strong potential benefits of the empowerment model, but it takes time and patience, she stressed.

Many examples of empowerment models, including participatory action research in adult literacy classes, have been documented since. Massachusetts has continued to support the training of Health Action Teams (Garner, 2008). In a recent empowerment model for health literacy, indigenous youth in British Columbia schools were assisted by university students to create videos on health topics of their choice (Stewart et al., 2008). The youth brainstormed ideas for health topics they thought were significant for themselves, and they came up with the following: drug and alcohol use, drinking and driving, diabetes, depression, sports, culture, seafood, the medicine wheel, colonization, dancing and singing, and fetal alcohol spectrum disorder. After making the videos they reported some healthy changes to their lives. One said that after making her video about traditional diets, she eats more seafood now realizing how healthy it is for her. Another said he intended to change his lifestyle with regard to alcohol and tobacco use and that it helped him stay out of trouble and in school. Others reported greater self-confidence as a result of their new skills and accomplishment with the video camera. The researchers described four 'metathemes' that developed through their data analysis: (i) community, (ii) culture, (iii) confidence, and (iv) control. They concluded that culture is central to Aboriginal health literacy, a point that Atleo makes clear in chapter 6 on Aboriginal peoples and health.

In another study on aboriginal health literacy (Antone & Ronson, 2009), seniors shared their understanding of health and its determinants and identified sharing cultural stories with aboriginal youngsters as a priority. This led to developing a project to 'empower' seniors to share cultural knowledge with children. Books by aboriginal authors and publishers that were appropriate for children learning to read were purchased. Seniors were driven to schools on a weekly basis to help aboriginal and other students read these books and learn more about their culture and about health from an aboriginal perspective.

Even when literacy programs do not directly address physical health issues, there is evidence showing positive health outcomes from literacy classes alone (Pignone, DeWalt, Sheridan, Berkman, & Lohr, 2005; Poresky & Daniels, 2001; READ Saskatoon, 2003). There is also evidence that seniors who volunteer as literacy tutors in schools experience less depression, more physical activity levels and stamina, higher mobility and flexibility, larger social networks, and better memory and executive function than other kinds of volunteers with similar demographics or those on a waiting list to become tutors (Tan, Xue, Li, Carlson, & Fried, 2006; Washington University, 10 March 2009).

Developing Ongoing Partnerships between
Health Agencies and Educational Institutions

In an extensive study of the delivery of a health curriculum for literacy learners in New York, called Study Circle+, one of the most important outcomes was the ongoing relationship that developed between the literacy centers and local health care institutions through this work. According to the project manager, the partnering is necessary so that health staff are not asked to come in for their content expertise on an ad hoc basis but through a continuing, dynamic relationship. As the health provider talks to the students, he or she gains knowledge that can be taken back to the hospital setting. This includes insights into issues that affect this population and about the barriers put up by the health system (Lawrence & Soricone, 2005). For example, students at the Mid-Manhattan Literacy Center were taken on a hospital tour, met with hospital department heads, and later gave feedback to hospital administration on how to improve the signage to make it more accessible for patients with lower literacy skills. Students also helped pilot test written educational materials, and the hospital improved their image in the community through working with the students.

What emerged from the original partnership was much more than teaching about low-cost health insurance or establishing a health literacy resource center, which were original goals. Other initiatives continue to be developed in New York, such as literacy fellowships provided to first year medical students to spend a term teaching literacy at the literacy centers (Tassi & Ashraf, 2008). As well, five hospitals there have now used volunteers trained to help people improve their health literacy in waiting rooms through a program developed in conjunction with a television channel devoted to adult learning and literacy (http://www.TV411.

org). In Canada, a similarly creative partnership developed between the Centre for Literacy Quebec and Montreal General Hospital (Centre for Literacy Quebec, 2001).

Building and strengthening such partnerships between schools and health institutions has proven to be beneficial in public schools as well. As an example, many schools in Ontario now have health action teams or healthy school committees that meet regularly with local public health staff and other community partners. These groups collaboratively assess and address health issues at the school with a focus on physical and social environments, policies, community services, and partnerships, as well as student health knowledge and behaviour, often starting with healthy nutrition and more time for physical activity both during instructional and extra-curricular time. Some agencies, such as the Canadian Lung Association, that have long provided programming for schools, now present their tobacco prevention curriculum within a Healthy Schools approach, and actively encourage the formation of school health action teams to work on initiatives that address the physical and social environments as well as instructional programming (The Lung Association, 2008, p. 4).

This form of partnering can be traced to ideas from the field of health promotion, particularly to the 'settings' approach to health promotion that has gained ground over health issue-specific starting points since the Ottawa Charter (WHO, 1986) and to the successes in Europe with multi-sectoral collaboration for health in the Healthy Cities initiative, and in the Health Promoting Schools (HPS) movement. HPS requires health-education partnerships from the highest level of national government as well as at the local level, which has led to partnership of nurses and doctors in many schools and the formation of school health teams and advisory committees to guide continuous programming.

In Ontario, as well as in many other provinces and countries, this work has been very important since it has provided a balance that many educators have found necessary to improve the lives and achievement of students who may be at risk in an environment where literacy and numeracy achievement testing is the primary focus. Such a narrow focus is suspected by many education scholars to be detrimental, since some students begin to view their language as substandard and themselves as inadequate compared to their peers based on continual assessment of these measures (Corbett, 2004). The achievement of students, then, can only be improved by more inclusive and broad-based activities that address social, emotional, mental, and physical health in a culturally meaningful way.

Implications for Research and Action

Professionals trained in medicine, nursing, and community health can continue to play an important role supporting efforts to improve literacy achievement *through improving health,* with research documenting that a Comprehensive School Health approach is indeed an effective strategy for literacy achievement as well as chronic disease prevention (Guertin, 2007). Many educators have been pleased, for example, that with the influence of those in the health sector, the Ministry of Education in Ontario has adopted and disseminated a Foundations for a Healthy School framework which helps balance literacy with health goals in schools; and many public health nurses are equally pleased that the Ontario Standards for Public Health now require them to collaborate with schools through an ongoing Healthy Schools approach.

As well, health and education professionals can continue to address health literacy through the development of plain language and multimedia resources on health topics, and through instructional programs to address these topics. They can advocate for adult education and literacy programs for their benefits to health as well as to education, and they can continue to collaborate with each other through the incorporation of health content and health literacy skills through such programs. Researchers in both fields need to continue to evaluate new initiatives and find and disseminate evidence for what works, so that new programs and initiatives can continue to be developed and improved for the well-being of present and future generations.

Suggestions for Teaching and Learning

We recommend that instructors challenge students to consider these follow-up activities:

1 Compare and contrast definitions of 'health,' 'health literacy,' and 'literacy' you can find in the academic literature. Why can't people agree about them?
2 If you are a health professional, team up with an educator and brainstorm projects that might serve both of your mandates or clientele within a 'settings' approach. Write a funding proposal for the best

idea, including Goal, Objectives, Rationale, Literature review, Work plan, Budget, and Evaluation plan.
3 Measure the readability level of a health information brochure or web-page, and rewrite it using a 'plain language' guide you can find on the Internet. Measure it again and see if you have improved readability.

REFERENCES

Antone, E., & Ronson, B. (2009). *Towards a meaningful definition of health literacy in the aboriginal community, Phase II: The 'Seniors' Aboriginal Literacy Project' – Aboriginal seniors tutoring elementary school children in Toronto* [Report]. Toronto: OISE/University of Toronto.

Baker, D.W., Parker, R.M., Williams, M.V., Clark, W.S., & Nurss, J. (1997). The relationship of patient reading ability to self-reported health and use of health services. *American Journal of Public Health, 87,* 1027–1030.

Baker, D.W., Gazmararian, J.A., Williams, M.V., Scott, T., Parker, R.M., Green, D., et al. (2002). Functional health literacy and the risk of hospital admission among Medicare managed care enrollees. *American Journal of Public Health, 92*(8), 1278–1283.

Baker, D., Wolf, M.S., Feinglass, J., Thompson, J.A., Guzmararian, J.S., & Huang, P. (2007). Health literacy and mortality among elderly persons. *Archives of Internal Medicine, 167*(14), 1503–1509.

Canadian Council on Learning. (2007). *Health literacy in Canada: Initial results from the international Adult Literacy and Skills Survey.* [Report]. Ottawa: Canadian Council on Learning.

Canadian Council on Learning. (2008). *A healthy understanding: What have we learned about health literacy in Canada?* [Report]. Ottawa: Canadian Council on Learning.

Canadian Public Health Association. (n.d.). Plain language service, frequently asked questions. Retrieved 15 January 2010 from http://www.cpha.ca/en/pls/faq.aspx.

Centre for Literacy Quebec. (2001). Health literacy project, Phase 1: Needs assessment for the health education and information needs of hard-to-reach patients. Retrieved 29 July 2009 from http://www.centreforliteracy.qc.ca/health/finalsum/bd/bdcover.html.

Clement, S., Ibrahim, S., Crichton, N., Wolf, M., & Rowlands, G. (2009). Complex interventions to improve the health of people with limited literacy: A systematic review. *Patient Education and Counseling, 75,* 340–351.

ContinYou. (2010). Skills for health. Retrieved 15 January 2010 from http://www.continyou.org.uk.

Corbett, M. (2004). Knowing a duck from a goose: The real world of education in an age of smoke and mirrors. *Our Schools/Ourselves, 13*(2), 95–122.

Corrigan, M., Bodane, C., & Rischbieter, R.G. (1994). *Health promotion for adult literacy students: An empowering approach. Alcohol and other drugs: Realities for you and your family.* Hudson River Center for Program Development, Inc.; University of the State of New York; State Education Department.

Critchley, M. (Ed.). (1978). *Butterworths medical dictionary.* London: Butterworths.

Garner, B. (2008). Literacy students as health advisors. *Focus on Basics: Connecting Research and Practice, 9* (B), 10–14.

Guertin, M. (2007). *An examination of the effect of a comprehensive school health model on academic achievement: The effect of living school on EQAO test scores.* Toronto: Ontario Institute for Studies in Education/ University of Toronto.

Hohn, M.D. (1998). Empowerment health education in adult literacy: A guide for public health and adult literacy practitioners, policy-makers and funders. Retrieved 25 November 2009 from http://www.nifl.gov/nifl/fellowship/reports/hohn/HOHN.HTM .

Institute for Healthcare Advancement. (2009). A recap of plenary and selected breakout sessions, IHA's 8th Annual Health Literacy Conference, Thursday, 7 May 2009. A Breakthrough health literacy program: Empowering parents, benefitting children, improving the healthcare system. Retrieved 12 July 2009 from http://www.iha4health.org/default.aspx/MenuItemID/337/MenuGroup/_Health+Literacy+Conference.htm.

Kickbusch, I. (2007). *Invest in health literacy: Enabling choices for health in modern societies.* Presentation at International Union of Health Promotion and Education (IHUPE) Conference, Vancouver, 14 June. www.ccl-cca.ca.

Lawrence, W., & Soricone, L.A. (2005). Conversation with FOB: Learning how to teach health literacy. *Focus on Basics: Connecting Research and Practice, 8* (A), 33–38.

Levy, S., Rasher, S., Carter, S., Harris, L., Berbaum, M., Mandernach, J., et al. (2008). Health literacy curriculum works for ABE students. *Focus on Basics: Connecting Research and Practice, 9* (B), 33–39.

Lindau, S.T., Tamori, C., Lyons, T., Langseth, L., Bennett C.L., & Garcia, P. (2002). The association of health literacy with cervical cancer prevention knowledge and health behaviours in a multi ethnic cohort of women. *American Journal of Obstetrics and Gynecology, 186*(5), 938–943.

Lung Association, The. (2008). *Lungs are for life: Grade 8 module prototype test 2008–2009.* Supported through the Ontario Ministry of Health Promotion. The Lung Association.

McMillan, M. (2007). *A health literacy manual to create awareness about diabetes.* Lunenburg, NS: Lunenburg County Adult Learning Network, Nova Scotia Department of Education.

Mossey, J.M., & Shapiro, E. (1982). Self-rated health: A predictor of mortality among the elderly. *American Journal of Public Health, 72*(8), 800–808.

Nielsen-Bohlman, L., Panzer, A., & Kindig, D.A. (Eds.). *(2004). Health literacy: A prescription to end confusion.* Washington, DC: National Academies Press.

Norton, M., & Horne, T. (1998). The wholeness of the individual: Linking literacy and health through participatory education. Retrieved 24 July 2009 from http://www.nald.ca/library/research/pat/245_247/page245.htm.

Nutbeam, D. (2000). Health literacy as a public health goal: A challenge for contemporary health education and communication strategies into the 21st Century. *Health Promotion International, 15,* 259–267.

Petch, E., Levitt, N., & Levitt, A. (2004). People who rate: Community involvement in the development of health education materials and messages. Presentation delivered to the Second Canadian Conference on Literacy and Health, Ottawa. October 2004.

Pignone, M., DeWalt, D.A., Sheridan, S., Berkman, N., & Lohr, K.N. (2005). Interventions to improve health outcomes for patients with low literacy: A systematic review. *Journal of General Internal Medicine, 20,*185–192.

Poresky, R.H., & Daniels, A.M. (2001). Two-year comparison on income, education, and depression among parents participating in regular Head Start or supplementary Family Service Center services. *Psychological Reports, 88:* 787–796.

READ Saskatoon. (2003). READ Saskatoon (re) writing our futures project. Retrieved 24 July 2009 from http://www.nald.ca/litweb/province/sk/readsask/pubs/lithelth/cover.htm.

Ronson, B., & Rootman, I. (2009). Literacy and health literacy: New understandings about their impact on health. In D. Raphael (Ed.), *Social determinants of health: Canadian perspectives* (2d ed.). Toronto: Canadian Scholars' Press.

Rootman, I., & Gordon-El-Bihbety, D. (2008). *A vision for a health literate Canada: Report of the expert panel on health literacy.* Ottawa: Canadian Public Health Association.

Rootman, I., & Raeburn, J. (1994). The concept of health. In A. Pederson, M. O'Neill, & I. Rootman (Eds.), *Health promotion in Canada* (pp. 56–71). Toronto: W.B. Saunders.

Rootman, I., & Ronson, B. (2005). Literacy and health research in Canada: Where have we been and where should we go? *Canadian Journal of Public Health, 96*(Suppl. 2), 62–77.

Rudd, R.E., & Comings, J.P. (1994). Learner developed materials: An empowering product. *Health Education Quarterly, 21*(3), 33–47.

Rudd, R.E., Epstein Anderson, J., Oppenheimer, S., & Nath, C. (2007). Health literacy: An update of medical and public health literature. In J.P. Comings, B. Garner, & C. Smith (Eds.), *Review of Adult Learning and Literacy*. Vol. 7. Mahwah, NJ: Lawrence Erlbaum Associates.

Statistics Canada. (1994). International adult literacy survey. Retrieved 15 January 2010 from http://www.statcan.gc.ca/dli-ild/data-donnees/ftp/ials-eiaa-eng.htm.

Statistics Canada. (2003). Building on our competencies: Canadian results of the international *a*dult literacy and skills survey. Ottawa: Statistics Canada. Cat. no. 89-617-XIE. Retrieved 15 January 2010 from www.statcan.ca/english/freepub/89-617-XIE/89-617-XIE2005001.pdf.

Stewart, S., Riecken, T., Scott, T., Tanaka, M., & Riecken, J. (2008). Expanding health literacy: Indigenous youth creating videos. *Journal of Health Psychology, 13,* 180.

Sudore, R.L., Yaffe, K., Satterfield, S., Harris, T.B., Mehta, K.M., Simonsick, E.M., et al. (2006). Limited literacy and mortality in the elderly, *Journal of General Internal Medicine, 21,* 806–812.

Tan, E.J., Xue, Q.L., Li, T., Carlson, M.C., & Fried, L.P. (2006). Volunteering: A physical activity intervention for older adults – The Experience Corps Program in Baltimore. *Journal of Urban Health, Bulletin of the New York Academy of Medicine, 83*(5): 954–969.

Tassi, A., & Ashraf, F. (2008). Health literate doctors and patients. *Focus on Basics: Connecting Research and Practice, 9* (B), 1–7.

UCLA Anderson School of Management [Press release, November 2007]. Retrieved 12 July 2009 from http://www.iha4health.org/default.aspx/MenuItemID/337/MenuGroup/_Health+Literacy+Conference.htm.

United States. Congress. House Committee on Education and Labor. (1991). National Literacy Act. Washington, DC: U.S.G.P.O.

Washington University, St. Louis. [Press release, 10 March 2009]. Studies show that students aren't the only ones who benefit from school-based tutoring. Retrieved 27 July 2009 from http://gwbweb.wustl.edu/newsroom/PressRelease/Pages/ExperienceCorpsEvaluation.aspx.

World Health Organization. (1946). Constitution. Geneva: WHO. Retrieved 15 January 2010 from www.who.int/governance/eb/who_constitution_en.pdf.

World Health Organization. (1986). Ottawa charter for health promotion. Ottawa: Canadian Public Health Association.

World Health Organization. (2005). Bangkok charter for health promotion. Geneva: WHO.

Zarcadoolas, C., Pleasant, A., & Greer, D.S. (2005). Understanding health literacy: An expanded model. *Health Promotion International, 20,* 195–203.

8 Women's Health and Learning: Working with Women Who Use Substances

DONNA M. CHOVANEC
AND BRETTANY JOHNSON

I am kind of *learning* that it's easier to face [my emotions] and deal with them than run away and cover them up and make them 10 times worse … So I'm *learning* to, I guess, deal with stuff.

> – woman in addictions outreach program of the Alberta Alcohol and Drug Abuse Commission (AADAC, 2006, p. 79)

As this volume makes abundantly clear, health and education are intricately linked on many dimensions. Both health promotion and health education recognize that a complex relationship among social factors – including education and literacy – affects health and vice versa. According to UNESCO (1997, p. 5), 'Adult education offers significant opportunities to provide relevant, equitable and sustainable access to health knowledge.'

Women's health experiences are of particular concern because women the world over are the informal health care providers and health care knowledge holders for their families and communities, yet they have the least access to health care resources and information (World Health Organization, 2009). In this chapter, we take a closer look at one particular health scenario – women and substance use – through which we analyse women's experience of the health and education nexus. Although substance abuse is only one example of the many ways in which women encounter the health and education systems, contemporary perspectives about women and substance use in Canada signal the kinds of linkages between health and education for women that we discuss in this chapter (Greaves & Poole, 2007; Health Canada, 2006).

In the first section, we ground our discussion of education and health by first describing the complex and marginalizing social context within which women's experiences of substance use are situated. We then make some general linkages between education/learning and women's substance use, followed by a more explicit connection between two inter-related treatment approaches that are recommended in the addictions literature – stages of change and motivational interviewing – and how learning might be understood to occur within these treatment processes. In this analysis, we explore key adult education concepts evident in experiential, transformative, and relational learning theories. These concepts are central to many chapters in this book, especially those of Ziegahn; Brookfield; and Kinsella, Caty, Ng, and Jenkins.

Our intent is to draw attention to the important educational work in the practice of counsellors, mental health professionals, support workers, and other service providers who are engaged in teaching-learning processes with women as they negotiate their experiences of substance use and make changes in their lives. In this chapter we spotlight women and substance use. However, our analysis will be useful not only for those who work with women in the addictions field but also for a broad range of service providers who interact with women in a diverse array of settings.

Women and Substance Use: Considering the Context

It is a well-known maxim in most helping professions to 'start where the person is' and then go from there. This requires sensitivity and understanding of the client's, patient's, or student's particular individual and social circumstances. In helping practices that acknowledge the role of context – for example, the determinants of health approach – there is an acute understanding of the importance of social and economic factors that contribute to health and educational status.

In this section, we consider the complex social, economic, and cultural contexts within which women's use of substances is located. In subsequent sections, we will address the relationship of this social context to their learning and educational experiences.

Until quite recently, our knowledge about substance use and about people who use substances was almost entirely based on men's experience and assumed to be equally applicable to women. Yet, women's experience differs significantly from that of their male counterparts. In addition to physiological differences, a particular constellation of social factors is especially relevant in women's experiences of substance use.

Demographically, women in treatment for substance use are younger and have lower incomes and educational levels than men – both of the latter are highly correlated with health status. There is a stronger influence of partners and family history in the trajectory of women's substance use, and women are more likely to have health and family problems (AADAC, 2006). Women with substance use issues are very likely to have been abused (Brown, 2008, June) and often face concurrent health problems, eating disorders, or post-traumatic stress (Greaves & Poole, 2007). As the primary caregivers, often as single parents, marginalized women face issues related to parenting more often than do men. Parental responsibilities include juggling the needs of children with attendance at health or educational programs, especially when unforeseen problems arise (AADAC, 2006; Chovanec & Lange, 2009). Child protection agencies often equate mothers' use of substances with child neglect or abuse, making it difficult for women to connect with community services for fear of losing their children (Boyd, 2007).

The complex interrelationship among these multiple social factors speaks to the general marginalization of women in society. In a spiraling process, as a woman is increasingly relegated to the margins of society, the factors that marginalize her then act as interlocking barriers in all aspects of her life, affecting her access to health care and education. Such a 'web of intersecting barriers' is described in a recent assessment of the learning and educational needs of marginalized adults in Edmonton (Chovanec & Lange, 2009, p. 94). The authors state:

> The most important finding is not related to the *individual* elements but rather, how these elements *interact*. Participants alerted us to the critical significance of understanding their life stories and social circumstances holistically, including how limited resources, parental responsibilities, lack of stability and support, learning issues and traumatic experiences are compounded to create a substantial barrier to entering or to continuing in their educational programs. (p. 67)

Underlying and heightening the complexity of these many marginalizing factors is social stigma: 'Women abusing drugs are more likely to be stigmatized by society than men abusing drugs because their activities are considered to be 'doubly deviant' (UNIFEM, n.d., p. 1). Stigma and shame prevent women from seeking treatment and support of any kind (AADAC, 2006; Brown, 2008).

Although we are speaking about women collectively here, experiences of substance use are not the same for all women. Women who are poor have fewer resources and are more frequently under surveillance by authorities such as child protection and criminal justice departments (Boyd, 2007). Aboriginal women are directly targeted as 'at risk' in campaigns to prevent Fetal Alcohol Spectrum Disorder (FASD) (Salmon, 2007). Racialized women; rural women; Lesbian, Bisexual, Gay, Transgendered, and Queer (LBGTQ) women; younger or older women; and women with disabilities all face distinctive issues that affect their access to resources, their learning experiences, and how their substance use is perceived and addressed.

Responding to the Learning Needs of Women Who Use Substances

Such a complex constellation of factors in the lives of women who use substances demands responses from service providers that are sensitive to their life circumstances and critical of the structural conditions and constraints impinging upon their lives.

To begin with, this requires a *self-reflexive* approach to working and interacting with women in which we critically examine our own biases and beliefs. Brown (2008, June) demonstrates that dominant addictions discourses about abstinence are ingrained in program policies and treatment practices across Canada, leaving no real choice for women who might seek alternatives. Addictions discourses have long been laden with moralistic overtones that denigrate poor and racialized groups for their supposed lack of 'willpower.' 'As the clients have experienced,' reports AADAC (2006), 'maintaining a non-judgmental stance can be a struggle for service providers when dealing with women who use substances' (p. 109). Unless service providers – counsellors, nurses, social workers, teachers, physicians, and so forth – engage in critical self-reflection, we risk carrying such judgments into our relationships with women and victimizing them further.

Second, effective and caring treatment and prevention related to women who use substances require a *holistic, woman-centred* approach that validates the complexity and interrelatedness of education and health with other physical, social, psychological, spiritual, and structural factors. Such an approach 'looks at the woman as a whole person as opposed to just … [a woman] with an addiction' (AADAC, 2006, p. 110). This holistic stance is shared by health promotion and adult education practitioners.

In her multi-dimensional model for FASD prevention, Poole (2007) applies this approach at a societal level. She criticizes the child-centred focus of most FASD prevention initiatives and advocates instead for a woman-centred approach that attends to women's health within the broad spectrum of other social factors in their lives, and that treats the mother and child as an interconnected unit. The first level focuses on a healthy society for all women, making 'broad efforts to change health and social policy to address poverty, violence against women, discrimination and other factors that contribute to women's substance use' (p. 293). The second level advocates a network of community supports for all women of childbearing years. The third level envisions 'a coordinated infrastructure of perinatal care' targeted to 'women at high risk of having a child with FASD' (p. 296). An approach that incorporates such sweeping societal changes will be familiar to adult educators whose grounding in critical social theory motivates an 'unrelenting critique of social structures' and 'a vision of society that is socially responsible' (Scott, 1998, p. 186).

Thus, in recognizing that experiences of substance use are gendered, as well as raced and classed, and are embedded in a complex constellation of social factors, woman-centred – and learning-centred – approaches to prevention and treatment have evolved that consider personal, social, and structural levels of change.

Adult Education and Learning Experiences

We begin here with an example of a woman-centred addictions outreach program that successfully integrates learning and education into its approach. AADAC's Enhanced Services for Women (ESW) program in Alberta provides treatment and support services to pregnant women who use substances. The program recognizes the complexity of women's lives and acknowledges the multiple barriers they may encounter in accessing and successfully completing treatment. ESW service coordinators use an outreach approach to provide crisis intervention and counselling, refer women to appropriate programs within AADAC's service network, and act as a liaison with other community services. They also provide ongoing education to AADAC staff and community professionals about working with pregnant women.

Underlying many positive outcomes reported by women who have engaged with ESW – including reducing harm, stable housing, improved relationships, and breaking the cycle of violence – are stories of women's learning (AADAC, 2006). Learning occurs in several domains, including learning about one's self, about strategies, about services, and about self-advocacy. ESW service coordinators help women stay focused on their goals by teaching techniques for managing anger and anxiety, establishing schedules, dealing with triggers, and setting boundaries, as well as for gaining insight into their problems and monitoring their progress. Although many women in the program focus on their parental responsibilities, some also pursue educational and employment goals. From college certificate programs and university degrees to vocational training and work experience programs, women feel better about themselves and 'really turn their lives around' when their educational and employment barriers are addressed (p. 92).

This program is one of many that use an adult learning approach. In this section we focus on the specific learning and educational dimension of the experiences of women who use substances: that is, women's educational trajectory, the role of community agencies, the educational components in treatment and support programs, and the learning processes involved in treatment approaches.

Educational Trajectory. Women experiencing problems with their substance use often report difficulties in school and lower educational attainment. For example, in 2004, 56 per cent of all women in AADAC services and 67 per cent of the women in a specialized outreach program for pregnant women had not completed high school (AADAC, 2006). One of these women describes the interrelationship of substance use, legal, and educational troubles:

> My whole life I've used drugs, like since I was 12, and it got me into a lot of trouble, you know, with the law. I mean I had numerous charges. Well, theft charges, assault charges, stuff like that. I could never do school. I always got kicked out of one school or the other 'cause I'd skip school. And then I'd just end up being expelled just because of the fact that I couldn't function because I was using. (p. 50)

Although some attend educational institutions for upgrading, certificate, or degree programs, adult women living on the margins of society often find *formal* education inaccessible and inflexible to their needs. Community-based, *nonformal* educational programs, such as adult literacy and pre-employment programs, are often more successful at reaching adults who are economically and socially marginalized (Chovanec & Lange, 2009).

The Role of Community Agencies

All community health and social services include education within their mandates. They provide *informal* education in the form of information pamphlets, individual counselling, or workshops on everything from nutrition, to parenting, to know-your-rights.

Many women who experience problems with their substance use engage with an extensive network of services. Primary care and community-based service providers are often in an advantaged position to conduct *screening* for substance use issues or engage in *early intervention* with women with whom they have an ongoing and trusting relationship (Health Canada, 2006). Brief interventions, such as motivational interviewing (to be discussed later), are useful in working with women early in the process of change. However, in screening for substance use, service providers must be 'sensitive to the varying literacy levels of clients' (p. 85).

Literacy educators can assist other service providers, including health practitioners and addictions counsellors, to design *literacy friendly* environments and adapt materials into clear language. The Northeast Edmonton Literacy Network is a collaborative effort to make it easier for adults with literacy challenges to access community resources. The Network's 17 agencies, including health and education services, are working together to increase awareness about literacy issues and improve their literacy practices.

Community *outreach* is vital in working with women who use substances; there are a plethora of community health, social service, and educational settings that could be targeted for information, education, and off-site service provision (AADAC, 2006; Health Canada, 2006).

Educational Components in Treatment and Support Programs

As is evident in Alberta's Enhanced Services for Women program described earlier, most therapeutic programs have clearly defined educational elements. Within gender-specific addictions programs, learning opportunities such as information sessions, life skills training, and skill-based workshops are integrated into the treatment routine to assist in developing knowledge and skills.

Notably, harm reduction is an inherently educational endeavour. Although rarely embraced in Canadian addictions programs, a harm reduction approach recognizes that abstinence is not an appropriate goal for all women (Brown, 2008, June). Instead, the focus for some women is on minimizing the harmful effects of substance use such as reducing the frequency of use, substituting substances, staying connected to services, and maintaining a healthy living environment (AADAC, 2006). Making these kinds of changes requires not only a counselling relationship but also one of teaching or coaching as the woman learns new information, knowledge, and skills, such as information about drugs and their effects, knowledge about the social circumstances of her substance use, and skills in advocating for relevant resources.

Therefore, it is important that addictions counsellors have not only well-developed counselling skills, but are also conversant in adult education principles as well as learning theories and models.

Learning Processes Involved
in Treatment Approaches

Processes of change are learning processes. In working with women who are experiencing problems related to their substance use, the integration of the 'stages of change' model and a closely related counselling approach – motivational interviewing – are the recommended best practices for facilitating the change process (Health Canada, 2006).

Prochaska and DiClemente's (1984) transtheoretical or 'stages of change' model recognizes that change is a process that occurs in stages over time, from having no intention to change, to considering the pros and cons of change, to making a decision and then acting on it, and, finally, self-efficacy in maintaining the change. A key assumption is that specific processes of change (e.g., consciousness-raising or self-re-evaluation) should be emphasized at specific stages to maximize the opportunity for successful change. 'Rather than focus on the problem (such as the substance use) and all the factors that reinforce it, this model focuses on the change process itself' (AADAC, 2006, p. 154).

The stages of change model is closely linked to motivational interviewing, a client-centred, semi-directed approach to counselling. The goal of motivational interviewing is to increase the individual's internal motivation to change by facilitating her own exploration and resolution of ambivalence (Miller & Rollnick, 2002). Four principles form the basis of the motivational interviewing approach: expressing empathy, developing discrepancy, rolling with resistance, and supporting self-efficacy. Each of these principles facilitates a learning process in which 'the counselor takes the role of interested teacher/guide who supports clients in learning about their options and strategies for change' (AADAC, 2006, p. 154).

Adult Learning Theories in Addictions Treatment Approaches

The field of adult education offers a rich intellectual tradition from which we can draw to explore the complex social nature of learning in the stages of the change/motivational interviewing approach. For our analysis, we draw on experiential, transformative, and relational learning theories.

Experiential learning theory is concerned with the way in which people interpret and internalize their everyday experiences to create new meaning. Jarvis's (1987) model is holistic and interactive and recognizes that people are contextually situated within a broader social, cultural world that informs the shape and scope of their experience. *Transformative learning* theory attends to the process by which adults make profound changes to their belief structures as a result of experience. According to Mezirow (1991), 'meaning perspectives' are the set of assumptions that influence how we perceive the world and interpret our experiences. 'Perspective transformation' occurs when an individual engages in a process of critical reflection that eventually prompts a fundamental transformation in her meaning perspectives.

Most learning models have limitations in terms of their ability to adequately conceptualize the nature of women's learning in substance use treatment because little work on women's learning has been undertaken (Flannery & Hayes, 2000). Therefore, we supplement this discussion by introducing *relational learning* concepts that figure prominently in theorizing about women's learning experiences (Flannery, 2000a) and in relational models that guide treatment with women (Finkelstein, 1996).

While not without criticism, relational-cultural theory (RCT) and self-in-relation theory have been most closely associated with integrated, gender-sensitive addiction treatment (Briggs & Pepperell, 2009; Finkelstein, 1996). These theories challenge models of human development that suggest healthy growth is characterized by the transition from dependence to independence (Jordan, 2010). Rather, theories of relationality suggest that women's development is situated within and contingent upon the development of relationships (Flannery, 2000a).

In the remainder of this section, we discuss three areas of congruence between the stages of change/motivational interviewing approach and our chosen learning theories: The role of disruption as an impetus for learning, the iterative and cyclical nature of learning and change, and a specifically gendered learning dimension.

Disruption plays a key role in prompting learning and change

Using the stages of change model is an effective way to work with women who are not ready to make a change in their substance use behaviour, thereby reducing the resistance that often accompanies treatment processes that move towards change too quickly (AADAC, 2006). While honouring the maxim that helpful counselling starts from where the individual is and respects the pace of her change process, the counsellor grounded in the motivational interviewing approach simultaneously helps the woman to increase her internal motivation for change and to move from one stage to the other.

In motivational interviewing, this is accomplished through uncovering 'discrepancies' by intentionally responding to client talk in a non-confrontational but directive manner that encourages 'cognitive dissonance' (Miller & Rollnick, 2002). This state of discomfort sets up a 'decisional balance' in which the client explores the benefits and risks of her substance use and the pros and cons of making changes. As the counsellor encourages the client to explore this tension, a tipping point may be reached, prompting personal learning that is a catalyst for change (Miller, 2005).

Key concepts from experiential and transformative learning theories help us to more fully explore the nature of the learning process prompted by discrepancies. For example, Jarvis (1987) suggests that learning is triggered by 'disjuncture' – the inability to understand, accommodate, or respond to a given situation by drawing on one's previous knowledge, beliefs, or skills. In an effort to resolve the disjuncture, the person engages in one or more cognitive, emotional, or action-oriented processes of learning that result in personal change. Mezirow (1991) similarly points to the role of a 'disorienting dilemma' as the basis upon which one begins to transform her meaning perspectives through critical reflection and dialogue with others.

By way of a simplified example, consider a discussion between a service provider and a pregnant woman who is using substances (disorienting dilemma). Employing a motivational interviewing approach, the service provider responds to the woman's concerns by offering information about the potential effects of different substances on the fetus (disjuncture). By intentionally enhancing the discrepancy between her desire for a healthy baby and the potential harmful effects of her substance use (decisional balance), the service provider facilitates a process of exploring the abusive experiences that have caused her to devalue herself and her body (a meaning scheme). As a result of this learning process, the client experiences increased resolve (motivation) to modify her behaviour by substituting a less harmful substance (new course of action), thereby protecting the health of her own body and that of her baby (perspective transformation).

By staying focused on the stage that the woman is experiencing *in the moment,* the service provider refrains from persuading or proscribing a course of action (such as abstinence) that may lead to resistance and reduce the probability of any change. Instead, she provides information that carefully heightens the woman's dissonance about her concerns, and then accepts her chosen course of action (harm reduction) (AADAC, 2006). Learning occurs as a result of the woman's *own* experience of disorientation, and at her own pace.

Thus, both experiential and transformative learning theories support a motivational interviewing approach, showing how disruption can act as a stimulus for personal learning and change in an ongoing process.

Learning and change is a cyclical and iterative process

Relapse or 'regression' is considered a normal part of the change process as individuals spiral or cycle through the stages (Prochaska & DiClemente, 1984). Our understanding of this iterative and cyclical process can be enhanced by drawing on experiential and transformative learning concepts to further explain how learning occurs *within* each stage, how a learning experience prompts movement *between* stages, and the role of learning in the occurrence of relapse.

In terms of learning within each of the five stages, Jarvis's model highlights the interactive nature of experience, in which 'there is always a feedback mechanism in each aspect of learning as well as a progressive dynamic' (Jarvis, 2008, p. 560). Jarvis emphasizes the 'trial and error' aspects of learning, in which we make multiple attempts to test a new idea before it is fully integrated as personal learning that resolves the original disjuncture. This helps to explain how a change process such as consciousness-raising or self-re-evaluation occurs several times over within a stage before a woman is sufficiently motivated or ready to move to the next.

In understanding the movement between stages, transformative learning theory provides some assistance through Mezirow's (1991) concept of perspective transformation. As an individual critically reflects on a disorienting dilemma, such as losing her children, she may revise, sometimes radically, her previously held perspective about her substance use, prompting her passage into the next stage.

As an almost predictable part of the change process, relapse plays an important learning role. Women who relapse may do so for a variety of reasons, but this experience contributes to the knowledge base they bring to subsequent engagement in the treatment process. Here is an example from a recent study:

> One woman's story describes how her earlier learning was used to her advantage after a relapse. After being abstinent for a year with the help of ESW and other services, she relapsed when she moved out of the city and lost her support network ... [After returning to services], she says, 'I knew what I had to do. I knew what worked for me before and I had to learn it again. Because it worked so well before.' (AADAC, 2006, p. 57)

Thus, women 'may be relapsing but they're in a different place' (p. 57). Through such a process, a woman is 'learning, unlearning and relearning' who she is, how to value herself, and how to move forward (Flannery, 2000b, p. 54).

Women's learning is relational and interconnected

In this section, we consider three areas of congruence with the women-centred addiction practices identified earlier, and with relational learning concepts: The integration of trauma-informed approaches to treatment, the role of dialogue in learning, and the processes of developing women's voice and agency.

In recognizing that women's experiences with substance use are interwoven with experiences of abuse, *trauma-informed treatment models* for working with women have recently evolved. In addition to many other cognitive and emotional goals, such programs help women to build trust and community with other women so as to lessen isolation, and to build safe and healthy interpersonal relationships.

Consistent with a relational approach, *dialogue* is a key component of the transformative learning process. Brooks (2000) asserts that, specifically in the case of women learners, transformative learning occurs in the course of sharing one's narrative. Personal storytelling is a trust-based, relational process that allows for reflective integration of the cognitive, emotional, and spiritual aspects of experience. In motivational interviewing, the process of uncovering discrepancies is a dialogue between the woman and counsellor in which the counsellor avoids the temptation to argue or convince the woman. Instead, it is a 'respectful process where the counselor works hard to hear the client's story' (Miller, 2005, p. 209).

For women-centred practitioners, dialogue is instrumental in helping women to reclaim *voice and agency*. According to Hayes (2000), 'A key assumption ... is that women lose or deny their "true" voices in response to the oppressive nature of social and cultural expectations for women' (p. 95). She identifies three processes of voice in women's learning that will be familiar to addictions counsellors working with women.

'Voice as talk' refers to the way women use language in conversation, a key component of the learning process. Through talk, we demonstrate and receive affirmation for our ideas, abilities, and identities (Hayes, 2000, p. 80). Motivational interviewing includes elements of what Hayes would call 'rapport talk,' a relationship-oriented conversational style that plays a role in creating a safe and open environment within which women can express themselves without fear of judgment.

'Voice as identity' refers to how women's identity is reflected in what they say, in the ideas they express, and in the confidence they convey. The learning processes involved include naming previously unarticulated experiences, finding a voice through expressing changing identities, and reclaiming voice. Hayes (2000) contends, 'Viewing our identities and voices as continual works in progress may offer important opportunities for the transformation of limiting assumptions about and labels for who we are and how we can express ourselves' (pp. 99–100).

In acknowledging the political nature of learning, 'voice as power ... emphasizes women's development of a consciousness of their collective identity and oppression as women, and of the means to challenge this oppression' (Hayes, 2000, p. 80). This process demonstrates the fundamental intersection of personal and social transformation. According to Scott (1998), 'While the self in the person changes in dialogue and in action (self power, self-concept), it is fundamentally a social process that transcends an individualistic concern for knowing' (p. 184). Voice as power reminds us that both micro and macro level change is needed for any substantive change to occur (Briggs & Pepperell, 2009).

Leslie (2007) provides an example of the relational approach in a program called Breaking the Cycle in Toronto, in which a group of health and social agencies collaborated to develop a comprehensive, integrated service for pregnant women who use substances. Key to the new service is a focus on mutual, empathic, and respectful relationships – that include caring, love, and hope – between program staff and women clients. These relationships are nurtured in a safe environment that is not necessarily devoid of conflict, but that effectively provides a 'template' for negotiating relationships in the future. Facilitating relationships among the women and building working relationships among service providers are additional components of the program. Leslie concludes, 'The experience of a growth-promoting relationship . . . can be a transformative experience' (p. 239).

Through a variety of means – including incorporating trauma-informed treatment approaches, engaging in mutual dialogue, and facilitating women's voice and agency – relational learning theories complement our understanding of the processes involved in woman-centred substance abuse treatment approaches.

Conclusion

In this chapter, we engaged the example of women and substance use to investigate the relationship between health and education for women. After reviewing the marginalizing contextual factors in the lives of women who use substances, we discussed the importance of responding with a self-reflexive, holistic, woman-centred, and critical approach to policy and practice. Then, starting from some general observations about the relationship of education/learning to substance use, we analysed the learning dimension of the stages of change model and motivational interviewing, highlighting elements of experiential, transformative, and relational learning theories.

We conclude with some examples about the applicability of our analysis to a variety of health and educational contexts.

First, although often ignored in health and educational contexts, the contextual factors of people's lives are germane to how and why they access, engage with, and benefit from health care and education. Furthermore, both poor health and low literacy are directly related to a complex constellation of societal factors and structural barriers. A critique of these conditions obliges adult educators and health practitioners to work for changes in the way social organizations are structured (Chovanec & Foss, 2006; Chovanec & Lange, 2009).

Second, the holistic, woman-centred approach to substance use reminds us to be mindful of difference, diversity, and uniqueness, not only in relation to gender but also in terms of race, ethnicity, culture, age, ability, sexuality, and so forth. For example, we might consider: What would an indigenous-centred approach to healthcare – one that was reflective of indigenous ways of knowing and healing – look like? We look with interest at what Atleo has to say about indigenous health in chapter 6 in this book.

Third, motivational interviewing is used for a variety of health issues beyond substance use, such as those for weight management and eating disorders. Rather than relying on rational argument, information, and persuasion, motivational interviewing in combination with the stages of change model provides a non-judgmental, systematic approach for recognizing and respecting individual readiness for change and assisting individuals to move from where they are to where they want to be (e.g., in their eating behaviour) at their own pace.

As our examples illustrate, education and health are intimately intertwined in the lives and experiences of us all. Our spotlight on women who use substances is instructive of the particular challenges and experiences of women who negotiate their health and learning in courageous and inspiring ways every day.

REFERENCES

AADAC. (2006). *Women working towards their goals through AADAC enhanced services for women (ESW): Technical report.* Edmonton, AB: AADAC.

Boyd, S.C. (2007). Introduction: The journey to compassionate care. In S.C. Boyd & L. Marcellus (Eds.), *With child: Substance use during pregnancy, a woman-centred approach* (pp. 10–19). Winnipeg, MB: Fernwood Publishing.

Briggs, C.A., & Pepperell, J.L. (2009). *Women, girls, and addiction: Celebrating the feminine in counseling treatment and recovery.* New York: Routledge.

Brooks, A.K. (2000). Transformation. In E. Hayes, D.D. Flannery, A.K. Brooks, E.J. Tisdell & J.M. Hugo (Eds.), *Women as learners: The significance of gender in adult learning* (pp. 139–153). San Francisco: Jossey-Bass.

Brown, C. (2008, June). It's not cut & dry: Women's experiences of alcohol use, depression, anxiety & trauma [PowerPoint slides]. Unpublished manuscript.

Chovanec, D.M., & Foss, K.M. (2006). Adult education and health: Will words get in the way? In T. Fenwick, T. Nesbit, & B. Spencer (Eds.), *Contexts of adult education: Canadian perspectives* (pp. 218–227). Toronto: Thompson Educational Publishing.

Chovanec, D.M., & Lange, E. (2009). *Beyond barriers: Maximizing access to learning for marginalized adults in the city of Edmonton*. Edmonton: University of Alberta.

Finkelstein, N. (1996). Using the relational model as a context for treating pregnant and parenting chemically dependent women. *Journal of Chemical Dependency Treatment, 6*(1), 23–44.

Flannery, D.D. (2000a). Connection. In E. Hayes, D.D. Flannery, A.K. Brooks, E.J. Tisdell & J. M. Hugo (Eds.), *Women as learners: The significance of gender in adult learning* (pp. 111–117). San Francisco: Jossey-Bass.

Flannery, D.D. (2000b). Identity and self-esteem. In E. Hayes, D.D. Flannery, A.K. Brooks, E.J. Tisdell & J.M. Hugo (Eds.), *Women as learners: The significance of gender in adult learning* (pp. 53–78). San Francisco: Jossey-Bass.

Flannery, D.D., & Hayes, E. (2000). Women's learning: A kaleidoscope. In E. Hayes, D.D. Flannery, A K. Brooks, E.J. Tisdell, & J.M. Hugo (Eds.), *Women as learners: The significance of gender in adult learning* (pp. 1–22). San Francisco: Jossey-Bass.

Greaves, M., & Poole, N. (Eds.). (2007). *Highs and lows: Canadian perspectives on women and substance use*. Toronto: Centre for Addiction and Mental Health.

Hayes, E. (2000). Voice. In E. Hayes, D.D. Flannery, A.K. Brooks, E.J. Tisdell & J.M. Hugo (Eds.), *Women as learners: The significance of gender in adult learning* (pp. 79–109). San Francisco: Jossey-Bass.

Health Canada. (2006). *Best practices – early intervention, outreach and community linkages for women with substance use problems*. Ottawa: Government of Canada.

Jarvis, P. (1987). *Adult learning in the social context*. London: Croom-Helm.

Jarvis, P. (2008). Religious experience and experiential learning. *Religious Education, 103*(5), 553–567.

Jordan, J. (2010). Recent developments in relational-cultural theory. In J. Jordan (Ed.), *The power of connection: Recent developments in relational-cultural theory* (pp. 1–4). New York: Taylor and Francis.

Leslie, M. (2007). Engaging pregnant women and mothers in services: A relational approach. In N. Poole & L. Greaves (Eds.), *Highs and lows: Canadian perspectives on women and substance use* (pp. 239–248). Toronto: Centre for Addiction and Mental Health.

Mezirow, J. (1991). *Transformative dimensions of adult learning*. San Francisco: Jossey-Bass.

Miller, G.A. (2005). *Learning the language of addictions counseling* (2d ed.). New York: John Wiley.

Miller, W.R., & Rollnick, S. (2002). *Motivational interviewing: Preparing people for change* (2d ed.). New York: Guildford Press.

Poole, N. (2007). A women-centred framework for the prevention of fetal alcohol spectrum disorder. In N. Poole & L. Greaves (Eds.), *Highs and lows: Canadian perspectives on women and substance use* (pp. 289–298). Toronto: Centre for Addiction and Mental Health.

Prochaska, J.O., & DiClemente, C.C. (1984). *The transtheoretical approach: Crossing traditional boundaries of therapy.* Homewood, IL: Dow Jones-Irwin.

Salmon, A. (2007). Beyond shame and blame: Aboriginal mothers and barriers to care. In N. Poole & L. Greaves (Eds.), *Highs and lows: Canadian perspectives on women and substance use* (pp. 227–235). Toronto: Centre for Addiction and Mental Health.

Scott, S.M. (1998). An overview of transformation theory in adult education. In S.M. Scott, B. Spencer, & A.M. Thomas (Eds.), *Learning for life: Canadian readings in adult education* (pp. 178–187). Toronto: Thompson.

UNESCO. (1997). The Hamburg declaration on adult learning: The agenda for the future. *Report from the Fifth International Conference on Adult Education.* Hamburg, Germany: CONFINTEA V.

UNIFEM. (n.d.). *Women and drugs: From hard realities to hard solutions (UNIFEM gender fact sheet no. 6).* Unknown: United Nations Development Fund for Women.

World Health Organization (WHO). (2009). *Women and health: Today's evidence tomorrow's agenda.* Geneva, Switzerland: WHO Press.

PART III

Educating Health Care Professionals

9   Teaching for the Health Professions

STEPHEN BROOKFIELD

This chapter explores the question: What do health education teachers need to know about teaching and learning to do good work? I try to answer this by drawing on knowledge from the general field of teaching and learning regarding what we know about student learning in general. I also consider a particular form of thinking employed by health professionals – clinical reasoning – and consider how this can best be taught. As I explore these two themes I am aware that the kind of learning people do around health behaviours, the knowledge that practitioners and patients need to acquire regarding health, and the barriers and constraints that the health system itself erects to inhibit learning are enormously complex and diverse. A renal dialysis technician, a pharmacist, and an occupational therapist work in very different settings, yet all need to explain information to others (colleagues and patients) in ways that are understood. In trying to ensure that people understand information as clearly as possible, these professionals are in fact working as teachers. This attention to good teaching practice is a theme for many of the writers in this book, including Pratt, Sadownik, and Jarvis Selinger; and Kinsella.

Given the particularity of health professionals' work, anything I write here should be taken with a healthy grain of salt (which, of course, is not healthy at all!). Learning tasks, learning settings, learners, and teachers themselves vary enormously, and it is a fool who claims to have found a set of generic behaviours that can be applied in a standardized way across all the contexts of health education. However, I do believe that it is worthwhile to consider general principles of teaching for the health professions. Principles can be malleable and manifest themselves differently in different situations. For example, we might hold the principle that learners should be treated respectfully; but what that looks like in practice will depend on many things, not the least of which are the cultural backgrounds of the learners and teachers involved.

General Principles of Teaching

In surveying the voluminous literature on principles of good teaching (Bain, 2004; Filene & Bain, 2005; McKeachie & Svinicki, 2004; Nilson, 2007; Weimer, 2003) it is easy to be diverted or bedazzled by key pedagogic characteristics or effective behavioural traits that can be incorporated into our practice. I am wary of objectifying the notion of good practice so that it becomes a set of standardized replicable behaviours. I believe that skillful teaching is a highly variable process that changes depending on any number of contextual factors. What does remain constant about skilful teaching is its being grounded in three core assumptions. How these assumptions frame practice varies enormously with the specific contexts of teaching, but their applicability holds true across diverse situations. These three core assumptions are that: (a) good teaching is whatever helps students learn, (b) the most effective teachers adopt a critically reflective stance towards their practice, and (c) the most important knowledge skilful teachers need to do good work is a constant awareness of how students are experiencing their learning and perceiving teachers' actions.

It also seems that students, whatever their age, wish to be treated as adults. They don't like to be talked down to or bossed around without reason. They don't trust (at least not initially) teachers who tell them that they (the students) know as much as the teacher and that everyone is an equal co-learner and co-teacher. To use Freire's terms (Horton & Freire, 1990) they want their teachers to be authoritative, not authoritarian. Nursing students know that their instructors have enormous experience and expertise that they (the students) don't have, and to pretend otherwise is inauthentic not to say dishonest. Adult students also say they wish to be treated with respect, though what that looks like varies enormously according to learners' class, race, and culture. One of the most important indicators they mention that convinces them they are being treated respectfully is the teacher attempting to discover, and address seriously, students' concerns and difficulties.

Students also want to believe that teachers know what they're doing, that they have a plan guiding their actions, and that they're not new to the classroom. They want to be able to trust teachers to deal with them honestly, and they hate it when they feel the teacher is keeping an agenda or expectation concealed from them. They like to know their teachers have lives outside the classroom, but they dislike it when teachers step over that line and make inappropriate disclosures regarding their personal life. They also want to be sure that whatever it is they are being asked to know or do is important and necessary to their personal, intellectual, or occupational development. They may not be able to understand fully and completely why the learning they are pursuing is so crucial but they need to pick up from the teacher the sense that this is indeed the case. One indicator of this that they look for is the teacher's willingness to model an initial engagement in the learning activity required. A preceptor who speaks out loud concerning her own clinical reasoning as she makes medical decisions is one who sets a tone for her students to do this. This kind of modelling is particularly appreciated where the learning involves a degree of risk and where failure entails (at least in the students' minds) public humiliation and embarrassment.

What Students Appreciate

In this section I want to explore the characteristics of helpful teachers that students say they particularly appreciate. In students' eyes an important component of successful learning is their perception of the teacher as both an ally and an authority. Students want to know their teachers stand for something and have something useful and important to offer, but they also want to be able to trust and rely on them. When describing teachers who have made a difference in their lives, or who are recalled as memorable and significant, students rarely speak the language of effectiveness. Instead they say they trust a particular teacher to be straight with them, or that a teacher really helped them 'get' something important.

A teacher is perceived as being effective because she combines the element of having something important to say or demonstrate with the element of being open and honest with students. Students do not measure a teacher's effectiveness solely in terms of a particular command of technique. Rather students want to feel confident they are learning something significant, and that as they are doing so they are being treated as adults. Given the diverse nature of North American society it is a mistake, in my view, to think we can generate the seven (or any other number) habits of effective teachers. Racial identity, learning style, personality, cultural formation, age, class location, gender, previous experience with the subject, readiness to learn, organizational values – all these factors and more render bland generalizations about effective teaching naïve and inaccurate. Working with Hmong patients is different than working with Somali students training to become respiratory therapists. Working as a primary care physician in an upper-class, white neighborhood will be different from working in a mobile health clinic in Compton, California.

Does this mean we are left with such a bewildering complexity of student identities, histories, and preferences that we simply throw up our hands and give up any hope of ever developing some broad guidelines to inform our teaching? Not necessarily. After reviewing thousands of critical incident questionnaires completed by students in different disciplines and geographic locations who represent a considerable diversity in terms of the factors identified above, it is clear that two general clusters of preferred teacher characteristics emerge. Both clusters are subject to multiple interpretations, and recognized in multiple ways, but both have enough internal validity to be considered useful guides to practice. These two clusters are credibility and authenticity.

Students define credibility as the perception that the teacher has something important to offer and that whatever this 'something' is (skills, knowledge, insight, wisdom, information), learning it will benefit the student considerably. Credible teachers are seen as those who exemplify such a high level of skilfulness that it is clear to students that they will learn something valuable from them. They are seen as possessing a breadth of knowledge, depth of insight, sophistication of understanding, and length of experience that far exceeds the student's own. Authenticity, on the other hand, is defined as the perception that the teacher is being open and honest in her attempts to help students learn. Authentic teachers do not go behind students' backs, keep agendas private, or double-cross learners by dropping a new evaluative criterion or assignment into a course half way through the semester. An authentic teacher is one that students trust to be honest and helpful. She/he is seen as a flesh and blood human being with passions, enthusiasms, frailties, and emotions, not as someone who hides behind a collection of learned role behaviours appropriate to the title 'professor.' From a student's viewpoint both credibility and authenticity need to be recognized in a teacher if that person is to be seen as an important enhancer of learning – as an authoritative ally, in other words. This holds true whether one is studying in a Bachelor of Pharmacy program or in a clinical setting in Community Health.

Interestingly, it appears that an optimal learning environment is one where both these characteristics are kept in a state of congenial tension. This holds true for online environments such as an online master's degree in health management just as much as for a face-to-face pharmacy rounds. A classroom where teacher credibility is clearly present but authenticity somewhat absent is one where students usually feel their time has been reasonably well spent (because necessary skills or knowledge have been learned), but also one that has been experienced as cold, unwelcoming, intimidating, or even threatening. Without authenticity the teacher is seen potentially as a loose cannon, liable to make major changes of direction without prior warning. Students often report a touch of arrogance or coldness about such a teacher that inhibits their learning. This creates a distance between teacher and learner that makes it hard for learners to ask for assistance, raise questions, seek clarification, and so on.

On the other hand, a classroom that is strong on teacher authenticity but weak on credibility is seen as a pleasant enough locale but not a place where much of consequence happens. Students often speak of such classrooms as locations to pick up easy grades and the teachers in charge as 'soft touches.' Authentic teachers are personally liked and often consulted concerning all manner of student problems. Students who feel they have been misunderstood or victimized by more hard-nosed teachers often turn to teachers they perceive as allies. The authentic teacher (Cranton, 2006) is seen as someone who will represent the student to the uncompromising teacher and convince unsympathetic colleagues that the student concerned has been misunderstood and is in fact a diligent learner. But being an advocate for a particular student is seen as something quite different than being an important learning resource. Students say that they like teachers they view only as authentic, but they don't usually stress how they learned something very important from them.

Emotional Rhythms of Learning

In this section I shift the focus from teaching to learning as I explore research into students' emotional responses to the experience of learning in higher education (Astin, 1997; Baxter Magolda, 1992; Evans, Forney, & Guido-DiBrito, 1998; King & Kitchener, 1994; Marton, Hounsell, & Entwistle, 1997; Pascarella & Terenzini, 1991; Perry, 1999: Weinstein, Palmer, & Hanson, 1995). Students rarely speak of learning in an emotionally denuded way. Developing understanding, assimilating knowledge, acquiring skills, exploring new perspectives, and thinking critically are activities that prompt strong feelings. This holds true across racial and gender differences as is evident in studies of African American, Hispanic, and Asian students (Cross, Strauss, & Fhagen-Smith, 1999; Gardella, Candales, & Ricardo-Rivera, 2005; Steele, 1995; Treisman, 1992) as well as work done on women's ways of knowing (Belenky, Clinchy, Goldberger, & Tarule, 1986; Belenky, Goldberger, Tarule, & Clinchy, 1996). Students talk about the exhilaration of intellectual stimulation, the anxiety of personal change, the pleasurable rush of self-confidence that comes from successful learning, and the shame of public humiliation that accompanies what they see as failure.

When students use the jargon of intellectual development to describe their learning journey they nearly always imbue it with emotional, even visceral, overtones. Physiological terms are invoked to describe moments of intellectual discovery or major breakthroughs in skill development. Learners talk of getting chills as they stumble across a piece of knowledge that puts everything into perspective, such as recognizing their own experience in Kubler-Ross's (1997) stages of dying or of painful knots of anxiety forming in their stomach as they fall short of self-imposed or teacher-prescribed standards. Some of the most emotionally laden themes are those concerned with self-doubts that are universally felt but rarely articulated. Students talk of feeling like an impostor, of committing cultural suicide, of losing the innocent belief that teachers have all the answers, and of regularly falling into demoralizing troughs of lost momentum. It is crucial for teachers to know how the emotional rhythms of these periods of self-doubt are experienced, because left untreated they may well end with the learner deciding she/he can no longer continue the journey. These emotions are silent killers of student engagement, a kind of pedagogic hypertension. On the surface students appear fine, yet internally they are experiencing emotions that can end their careers as learners. This chapter explores these emotions and considers how teachers might respond to these as they see them in students, colleagues, and patients across a range of health care settings.

Impostorship

Impostorship (Brookfield, 2006) is the sense learners report that at some deeply embedded level they possess neither the talent nor the right to become college or university students. Students who feel like impostors imagine that they are constantly on the verge of being found out, of being revealed as being too dumb or unprepared for college-level learning. The secret they carry around inside them is that they don't deserve to be a student because they lack the intelligence or confidence to succeed. They imagine that once this secret is discovered they will be asked to leave whatever program they happen to be enrolled in, covered in a cloud of public shame, humiliation, and embarrassment. Each week that passes without this event happening only serves to increase the sense that a dramatic unmasking lies just around the corner. 'Surely,' the student asks herself, 'sooner or later someone, somewhere is going to realize that letting me onto this campus was a big mistake. I'm not smart enough to succeed.'

Not all share this feeling, it is true, but it does seem to cross lines of gender, class, and ethnicity. It is also felt at all levels, from developmental, remedial learners to participants in doctoral seminars. The triggers that induce impostorship are remarkably predictable. One is the moment of being publicly defined as a student. Gardella et al. (2005) are typical when they write of the Latino/Latina adults they studied that 'deciding to go to college was itself a developmental crisis that challenged assumptions, expectations, and beliefs' (p. 43). The news that one has been admitted into an educational program is greeted by many applicants with a sense of disbelief, not entirely pleasurable. When students finally get to their first classes, their sense of impostorship is compounded by teachers asking all the participants to introduce themselves at the opening session and to talk about their previous experiences, current interests, and deepest enthusiasms. Teachers do this as a way of relieving students' anxieties and making them feel welcome. But this practice often seems to have the converse effect of heightening anxieties for many students. Rather than affirming and honouring their prior experiences, this round table recitation of past activities, current responsibilities, and future dreams serve only to convince such learners that everyone else in the class will make it while she/he will be the one person who just won't get it.

Expert teachers then ratchet up these feelings of impostorship to an almost unbearable level by telling students that they have to think critically about the new subject matter they are studying. Many students feel a reverence for what they define as 'expert' knowledge enshrined in professors' heads and academic publications. Being asked to undertake a critical analysis of ideas propounded by experts smacks of temerity and impertinence to them. They report that their own experience is so limited that it gives them no starting point from which to build an academic critique of major figures in their fields of study. There is a kind of steamroller effect in which the status of 'theorist' or 'major figure' flattens these students' fledgling critical antennae. In health promotion, for example, a diabetes educator or community dietician would hesitate to critique a health promotion expert.

Impostorship should be named and acknowledged early on by the educator. She can talk about how she felt like an impostor the first time she was asked to learn a particular technique or exercise a particular skill. Bringing working practitioners or former students to talk about the way they managed their own impostorship is always helpful. It is also important that a controlled sense of impostorship is a spur to further learning. Once a practitioner feels she is in such command of her field that no further study is necessary, then inertia begins.

Cultural Suicide

Cultural suicide describes the process whereby students are punished by their families, peers, and communities for what appears to be an act of betrayal; that is, to be seen to be changing as a result of participating in learning. This risk forces itself onto the consciousness of students of colour in high school, just as taking education seriously is condemned as 'acting White' (Bergin & Cooks, 2002). It is felt particularly keenly by students of all racial backgrounds who are first in their family to go to college or university and also by many adult learners. Cultural suicide is something that also affects working-class students who 'often become alienated from their families in direct proportion to their procurement of new ideas and attitudes' As a result they 'feel their identities shattered, and find themselves psychologically adrift' (Casey, 2005, p. 35). Students intuitively sense from their intimates and work colleagues that if higher education prompts them to begin a critical questioning of conventional assumptions and beliefs shared by these peers they (the students) will risk being excluded from the culture that has defined and sustained them up to that point in their lives. Just showing how much they are learning, growing, and changing, even if this involves no criticism of partners, friends, and colleagues, can be risky, leading eventually to cultural suicide. The perception of this danger, and experience of its actuality, is a common theme in working-class students' autobiographies (see, for example, Dews & Law, 1995; Welsch, 2004) and was even the topic of a successful commercial feature film, *Educating Rita*. Students who take critical thinking seriously and start to question shared assumptions, or students who clearly believe themselves to be changing for the better as a result of their learning, report that those around them start to view them with fear and loathing, with a hostility borne of incomprehension.

Health professionals can help prepare patients for cultural re-entry by suggesting ways to speak about their medical condition, history, or treatment using examples and language that are familiar and therefore understandable. Expecting patients to return to their families and speak as if they were professionals themselves places strain on both the patient and the family. So a liberal use of analogies and metaphors will be a crucial element in teaching health behaviours.

Lost Innocence

Students often come to campus with high hopes. They think that university or college will turn their lives around, that now they are going to get 'truth,' and that finally they'll understand how the world really works and who they really are. Going to university or back for a master's degree is viewed as a transformative marker event that's going to change their lives dramatically for the better by opening up career possibilities and helping them to self-knowledge. However, this sense of confidence is sometimes eroded almost from the first week as these students hear how their teachers describe learning, particularly in more social science-oriented programs in health such as Master of Public Health or Master of Hospital Administration. If professors stress that there are sometimes no right answers in clinical practice and that students will have to discover their own meanings for themselves, this can be disconcerting. When students ask teachers for the correct response regarding the application of a procedure or interpretation of data, and teachers reply 'it depends,' ... these same teachers then go on to say that knowledge and ideas cannot be understood in starkly dualistic terms, as either right or wrong. Instead, the world of intellectual inquiry is painted with the grey shades of ambiguity. Students are told that the purpose of a university or community college education is to get them to ask the right questions, not to find the right answers.

As students hear all this they sometimes feel cheated, lost, and confused. Or they just don't believe it. To them the professor is playing a sophisticated and evasive guessing game, pretending not to have the answer and testing the students to see if they have the wherewithal to push him to own up to the truth. When the penny drops and students realize their teachers mean what they say about there being no easy answers, universally correct views, or unequivocally right response to complex situations, they panic. This intellectual anxiety attack is a crucial one in students' autobiographies as learners. If they can live through it they experience an epistemological transformation. Knowledge and truth become seen as contextual and open, as constantly created and rec-reated in a community of knowers. Students realize their lives as learners will be marked by continual inquiry, questioning of assumptions, and reframing of perspectives, just as their teachers say it will. However, if students can't face this epistemological reframing, they are at a high risk of dropping out of the whole undergraduate experience.

A skilful teacher must strive to find ways of teaching students about the importance of context to health behaviour and the ways that each person's racial identity, cultural history, learning style – as well as their physiology or brain chemistry – affect how diagnoses are made and health protocols applied. This is a critical perspective that English develops in the opening chapter of this book. The skilful teacher, in using this approach, should try to alert students to the fact that political and community factors such as budget constraints or mistrust of how health agencies have acted in the past, need to be taken into account. One way to do this is constantly to bring into classrooms recent students who are now in the community or on the ward practising their skills and trying to deal with all the contex-tual factors the real world throws up in their face. Using recent graduates as experiential experts who can come back to the classroom and talk about their first months on the job brings home dramatically how newly minted health professionals need to adjust to context.

Roadrunning

As students speak about how they experience learning new skills, knowl-edge, and concepts they describe a rhythm that might be called incremen-tal fluctuation. Put colloquially, this learning rhythm can be understood as one where the learner takes two steps forward, one step back, followed by four steps forward, one step back, followed by one step forward, three steps back, and so on in a series of irregular fluctuations marked by over-all progress. It is a rhythm of learning that is distinguished by a gradually increased ability to learn new skills and knowledge juxtaposed with regu-lar interruptions and dissonances when it seems progress is impossible. When these apparent regressions to earlier ways of thinking and acting take place they are felt as devastatingly final. Instead of being viewed as the inconvenient interludes they really are, they seem like the end point of the process. In these moments of self-doubt students believe they will never 'get it,' that the learning concerned is 'beyond them,' and that they will therefore never become competent nurses or dieticians. They are tempted to return to tried and trusted ways of thinking on the grounds that even if these didn't always work or make sense at least they were familiar and comfortable.

The way this halting, jagged, incrementally fluctuating rhythm of learning is spoken of reminds me of the long-running Warner Brothers' Road Runner cartoon, where the same scene is repeated endlessly. The Road Runner is hurtling along the highway, his 'beep beep' cry raising Wile E. Coyote's frustration to ever-higher levels. The Road Runner comes to the edge of a canyon, and, because he's possessed of supernatural powers, he leaves solid ground to go out into mid-air. The coyote picks up his speed, and hurtles off the edge of the canyon into thin air in frantic pursuit, his legs pedalling in space. After about three seconds, however, the coyote realizes his situation. He freezes and looks down at the canyon floor several hundred feet below. Realizing the nature of his situation he plunges to the canyon floor and the screen is a mess of limbs and disconnected but bloodless body parts. In the next frame, of course, we see that the coyote has been magically reassembled off-camera and that the chase has begun anew.

Like the coyote, students often experience the beginnings of a new program with boundless energy and an optimistic sense of how it will make their lives better. Entranced by the prospect of transformation – of learning new skills and knowledge that will open new employment opportunities, bring self-knowledge, or help them develop self-confidence – they embrace the changes they know higher education entails. As they begin struggling to discard or reformulate assumptions and understandings that now seem not to explain the world adequately, there is a sense of forward movement, of progress towards true clarity of perception. But as students leave behind the solid ground of their old ways of thinking and acting, their enthusiasm sometimes turns to terror. They realize that they have nothing that supports them. Their previously solid and stable assumptive clusters and skill sets have evaporated, but no substitutes have solidified to take their place. This is the moment when their confidence drains away. They crash to the floor of their emotional canyons resolving never to go through this experience again.

Sooner or later, however, students are confronted by whatever hopes and dreams, or niggling anomalies or discrepancies, that spurred them to enroll in college or university in the first place. Learning begins anew, but this time students know that at some point they will find themselves perched precariously above the canyon floor. Out of such knowledge comes the ability to stay dangling for a few seconds longer than was formerly the case. There are, however, two things instructors can do. First, they can alert students to the fact that this rhythm is going to happen, so that when it does take place students don't think they are the only ones subject to this. Knowing this is a predictable, even normal, rhythm of learning can help students keep it in perspective. Second, teachers can do their best to structure classrooms for team and group work so that students develop small, supportive learning communities.

Community

Time and time again, as students speak about their crashing to the canyon floor, it becomes clear that the people who pick them up, dust them off, and set them back on track are their peers. The importance to students of belonging to an emotionally sustaining peer learning community cannot be overstated. 'Community' might seem a rather grandiose word to describe the clusters of four or five good friends that students say they value so highly. But the emphasis the members of these groups place on the emotional warmth and psychological security they provide makes the term 'community' more appropriate than, say, 'network.'

The important thing about these small communities is that they reassure their members that their private anxieties are commonly experienced. Through talking about their individual experiences of learning, students come to know that crashing to the canyon floor is a predictable moment not an idiosyncratic event. Learners lucky enough to be members of emotionally sustaining, peer learning communities speak of them as 'a second family' or 'the only people who really know what I'm going through.' These communities provide a safe haven, an emotional buttress against the lowest moments in their autobiographies as learners. Having a gallery of bios and photos, and links to each student's MySpace page, using group and team projects or presentations in class, or asking small groups of students to car pool as a way of getting to and from class are all things that help develop community.

Teaching Clinical Reasoning

Health education practice, as most practitioners know, is frequently located in a zone of ambiguity. The reality of clinical experience often stands in marked contrast to the patterns of practice laid out in introductory texts and pre-service education. In this section I want to argue that pre-service education still plays a crucial role in professional development, but only if pre-service curricula place the acquisition of the thinking skills of clinical reasoning at their centre. Such skills might be regarded as the meta-cognition of clinical practice. They shape the way practitioners approach, analyse, and respond to the multiple contexts and idiosyncrasies of practice. They do not displace the learning of specific skills or protocols, but they do frame how we determine the appropriateness of these protocols for different situations and how we modify the application of these skills in practice.

How can clinical reasoning best be taught? In interviews with practitioners the factor emphasized more strongly than anything else is their seeing it publicly modelled by figures of authority and power (Brookfield, 1995). When students see preceptors and allied health professionals speaking out loud the reasons for their decisions, or disclosing the cues they take seriously and how these help them construct ladders of inference, it becomes clear to novices how experts do clinical reasoning in field settings. Modelling can, of course, be done alone or in interprofessional teams, a focus of Gastaldi and Hibbert in this text. For many health educators the necessities of practice will mean this will happen in isolation, where one professional will attempt to model for students or novices her own engagement in clinical reasoning. But, since the clinical reasoning process depends so much on colleagues serving as critical mirrors, one of the most powerful forms of modelling is that undertaken in teams. If those perceived as credible experts demonstrate publicly how they rely on team colleagues to be their critically reflective mirrors, this sends a message to newly engaged practitioners that enlisting the help of colleagues is crucial to accurate clinical appraisal.

In my view, the importance of health education faculty undertaking a public modelling of their commitment to team learning cannot be emphasized too much. The more that faculty are publicly engaged in team teaching, team research, team writing, and team reflection on common problems, the more that they convey to practitioners an atmosphere that supports this. One reason it is important that faculty do this is because people often assume that good team behaviour means taking the reins and assiduously demonstrating their 'leadership' by speaking frequently, being the author and deliverer of team progress reports, and so on. It is important that practitioners learn early on that effective participation in teams does not boil down to talking a lot and being the person who writes, posts, and publicly reports the conversations a group is having.

When modelling team behaviours for students it is important that faculty show that interprofessional learning involves such things as: listening carefully, elucidating connections and links between different participants' contributions, showing appreciation for others' contributions, drawing others out through skilful questioning, calling for occasional periods of reflective silence, and being ready to speak one's mind in the face of new arguments or information. This is very close to the conditions of Habermas's ideal speech situation (Brookfield, 2004). Effective team participation sometimes also involves people arguing against the conventional wisdom and common sense explanations a group immediately adheres to, and insisting that certain ignored or discredited ideas and traditions be included. This is what Marcuse calls the practice of liberating tolerance in discussion (Brookfield & Preskill, 2005). For example, critical debate or the 'methodological belief' exercises ask participants to spend a limited time seeing a clinical situation from a viewpoint they may never have inhabited before – that of a patient, a patient's family member, or another specialist member of the medical team (anaesthetist, nutritionist, and so on).

Conclusion

I began this chapter by emphasizing the contextual, shifting nature of what we consider good practice. So perhaps it is appropriate to end it by acknowledging that although the situational nature of teaching cannot be denied, there are some broad insights we can hold on to. First, there are some definite similarities across learners of different ages, races, cultures, genders, and personality types regarding their perceptions of teachers. Credibility, authenticity, modelling, full disclosure, and consistency are some of the characteristics universally appreciated in teachers. There also seem to be some distinctive tensions and emotional rhythms experienced by very different groups of learners. Impostorship, cultural suicide, lost innocence, incremental fluctuation, and a yearning for community are all mentioned as being at the heart of the student experience. These characteristics, tensions, and rhythms have a level of generality that make them worthy of the attention of teachers in the health professions.

This chapter closes with a case developed by Carmen Hall, Mae McWeeny, and Stephen Brookfield that readers might use to apply some of the ideas in this chapter.

Orienting New Staff

Sue, R.N., is the orientation coordinator on a unit that is expecting five new hires in the first week of June. This will be the first orientation to occur in two years. The new hires will include one new ADN grad, two RNs with experience from other specialties, and two nursing assistants. In addition, a commitment was made earlier in the year to sponsor a nurse extern – a baccalaureate nursing student who has completed the third year of matriculation and will have an eight-week work experience on the unit.

Sue is excited about having new employees again. However, she believes this will be a challenge for the unit, which has historically been very busy in the summer. She has decided to prepare for the new employees arrival by revising the unit's orientation program. A review of evaluations completed by participants in previous orientations has led Sue to think that she can shorten the orientation process by one week. She believes that the shorter orientation period is more focused and that it permits earlier integration of the new staff members into the regular staffing pattern. Feedback from a regulatory visit suggested that the hospital could improve the documentation of employee competency. Therefore Sue has increased the number of validations that are to be documented by the preceptors.

Sue has recruited five colleagues to become new preceptors. She knows that preceptors usually need to work with the orientation program a few times before they feel confident about the process and documentation. Consequently, she has concerns about their inexperience. Therefore, in addition to her other preparations Sue has sent a letter to the staffing office to insist that the five preceptors be scheduled for the one-day workshop 'Precepting the Adult Learner' that is to be held in two weeks. This workshop has always served successfully as the orientation for new preceptors.

1 What assumptions do you think Sue is operating under as she prepares this orientation? List as many as you can.
2 Of the assumptions you've listed, which ones could Sue check by simple research and inquiry? How could she do this?
3 Give an alternate interpretation of this scenario. Develop a version of what's happening that is consistent with the events described but that you think Sue would disagree with.

We encourage students to work together to brainstorm these questions, not only to find answers but to establish further lines of inquiry and to create a springboard for further dialogue about teaching and learning in the health professions.

REFERENCES

Astin, A.W. (1997). *What matters in college: Four critical years revisited.* San Francisco: Jossey-Bass.

Bain, K. (2004). *What the best college teachers do.* San Francisco: Jossey-Bass.

Baxter Magolda, M. (1992). *Knowing and reasoning in college: Gender related patterns in student development.* San Francisco: Jossey-Bass.

Belenky, M.F., Clinchy, B.M., Goldberger, N.R., & Tarule, J.M. 1986. *Women's ways of knowing: The development of self, voice and mind.* New York: Basic Books.

Belenky, M.F., Goldberger, N.R., Tarule, J.M., & Clinchy, B.M., (1996). *Knowledge, difference and power: Essays inspired by women's ways of knowing.* New York: Basic Books.

Bergin, D.A., & Cooks, H.C. (2002). High school students of color talk about accusations of 'acting white.' *Urban Review, 34*(2), 13–34.

Brookfield, S.D. (1995). *Becoming a critically reflective teacher.* San Francisco: Jossey- Bass.

Brookfield, S.D. (2005). *The power of critical theory: Liberating adult learning and teaching.* San Francisco: Jossey-Bass.

Brookfield, S.D. (2006). *The skillful teacher: On technique, trust and responsiveness in the classroom* (2d ed.). San Francisco: Jossey-Bass.

Brookfield, S.D., & Preskill, S. (2005). *Discussion as a way of teaching: Tools and techniques for democratic classrooms* (2d ed.). San Francisco: Jossey-Bass.

Casey, J.G. (2005). Diversity, discourse, and the working-class student. *Academe, 91*(4), 33–36.

Cranton, P.A. (Ed.). (2006). *Authenticity in teaching: New directions for adult and continuing education,* # 111 (pp. 1–12). San Francisco: Jossey-Bass.

Cross, W.E. Jr., Strauss, L., & Fhagen-Smith, P. (1999). African American identity development across the life span: Educational implications. In R. Sheets & E. Hollins (Eds.), *Racial and ethnic identity in school practices* (pp. 29–47). Mahwah, NJ: Lawrence Erlbaaum Associates.

Dews, C.L.B., & Law, C.L. (Eds.). (1995). *This fine place so far from home: Voices of academics from the working class.* Philadelphia: Temple University Press.

Evans, N.J., Forney, D.S., & Guido-Di Brito, F. (1998). *Student development in college: Theory, research and practice.* San Francisco: Jossey-Bass.

Filene, J., & Bain, K. (2005). *The joy of teaching: A practical guide for new college instructors.* San Francisco: Jossey-Bass.

Gardella, L.G., Candales, B.A., & Ricardo-Rivera, J. (2005). 'Doors are not locked, just closed': Latino perspectives on college. *New Directions for Adult and Continuing Education, 108:* 39–51.

Horton, M., & Freire, P. (1990). *We make the road by walking: Conversations on education and social change.* Philadelphia: Temple University Press.

King, P.M., & Kitchener, K.S. (1994). *Developing reflective judgment: Understanding and promoting intellectual growth and critical thinking in adolescents and adults.* San Francisco: Jossey-Bass.

Kubler-Ross, E. (1997). *On death and dying.* New York: Scribner.

Marton, F., Housell, D., & Entwistle, N. (Eds.). (1997). *The experience of learning: Implications for teaching and studying in higher education* (2d ed.). Edinburgh: Scottish Academic Press.

McKeachie, W., & Svinicki, M. (2004). *McKeachie's teaching tips: Strategies, research, and theory for college and university teachers.* Florence, KY: Wadsworth.

Nilson, L.B. (2007). *Teaching at its best: A research-based resource for college instructors.* San Francisco: Jossey-Bass.

Pascarella, E.T., & Terenzini, P.T. (1991). *How college affects students: Findings and insights from twenty years of research.* San Francisco: Jossey-Bass.

Perry, W.G. (1999). *Forms of intellectual and ethical development in the college years: A scheme.* San Francisco: Jossey-Bass.

Steele, C.M. (1995). Stereotype threat and intellectual test performance of African Americans. *Journal of Personality and Social Psychology, 69*(5), 797–811.

Treisman, U. (1992). Studying students studying calculus: A look at the lives of minority mathematics students in college. *College Mathematics Journal, 23*(5), 362–372.

Weimer, M. (2003). *Learner-centered teaching: Five key changes to practice.* San Francisco: Jossey-Bass.

Weinstein, C.E., Palmer, D.R., & Hanson, G.R. (1995). *Perceptions, expectations, emotions and knowledge about college.* Clearwater, FL: H and H Publishing.

Welsch, K.A. (Ed.). (2004). *Those working Sundays: Female academics and their working class parents.* Lanham, MD: University Press of America.

10   Adult Learning in Public Health Nursing Practice

JANE MOSELEY

Integral to public health nursing practice is knowledge and application of adult learning theory that supports the transfer of information from the sciences of public health to individuals, families, groups, and populations. This chapter details 'why' this transfer occurs: to demonstrate evidenced-informed practice and accountability to meet the public health goals to protect, promote, and restore the peoples' health. The chapter also suggests 'how' this transfer might occur: through the author's Framework for Population-Focused Nursing Practice, a teaching framework which integrates adult learning concepts and principles with public health and nursing knowledge. Examples are given of how adult learning is integrated into public health practice and services. The Framework is applicable for maternal and child health programs such as prenatal classes and parenting classes; for communicable disease programs such as H1N1/flu immunization clinics, HPV and Hepatitis immunizations to school children; and for health promotion activities in schools and community such as community heart health programs, and community kitchens.

Defining Public Health

Often the terms used by health care professionals are confusing to the general population; indeed, even health professionals disagree on some terms. Perhaps the most challenging is finding a definition of public health that reflects the learner-centred nature of practice. Shah (2003) says that in Canada 'sometimes it [public health] refers to the publicly funded healthcare system' (p. 474), and at other times it refers to population health. Last (2001) agrees with the Milbank Memorial Fund

Commission Report of 1976 that public health is a social institution, a discipline and a practice (p. 145). In this chapter when I refer to public health I am referring to the social institution, the provincial and territorial institutions whose core functions are population health assessment, health surveillance, health promotion, disease and injury prevention, and health protection. After the 2003 SARS outbreak in Ontario, the federal government followed recommendations from the National Advisory Committee on SARS and Public Health (2003) and set up a national institution, the Public Health Agency of Canada (PHAC), to coordinate public health services between provinces and territories. Meanwhile, I use the broader term, 'community health nursing' for nursing practice, as this term includes public health nurses and home health nurses (Community Health Nurses Association of Canada (CHNAC), 2003). A focus on learning in the community is shared by many writers in this collection, including Ziegahn and Egan (chapters 3 and 4), both of whom write about strengthening community connections.

Public Health Nursing Context

My experiences in community health/public health nursing are from a Canadian context as an outpost nurse, a public health nurse, and currently as a university professor teaching community health to undergraduate nursing students whose clinical experiences are with community health services and programs. An important role for public health nurses is that of educator, to facilitate the transfer of health and disease information to individual clients, families, groups, communities, and populations.

Over the almost four decades since I became a nurse, there has been a gradual change in how public health nursing is practised. When I first graduated in 1972, 'patient teaching' was the term used for health education. Patient teaching included learning theories such as cognitive and behavioural approaches in order to teach patients about their normal body processes and/or conditions/diseases, with the overall goals of improving the health of the individual. The nurse was the expert with information to pass to the patient, the learner. My first work experience as an outpost nurse in northern Quebec quickly debunked this myth. I may have known about medical diseases, nursing interventions, and patient teaching but the people in the communities knew how to apply the knowledge in their reality context – how to survive, work, and stay healthy in the context of the harsh environment of wind and water, ice and snow. They knew much more about socio-cultural norms; family connections and relationships; availability of resources for diet, community supports, and medical aids; the impact of disease on quality of life; and death as a normal part of life. Although my nursing training prepared me to provide care and to teach individuals and families, my outpost nursing experience showed me I was a novice in health education in the context of community.

When I moved into the public health workforce in 1979, I realized that understanding and applying adult learning principles in health education was an expectation for public health nurses. Yet, the understanding of adults as individual learners and as a collective was limited. Adult learning generally meant relating 'principles' to group learning situations such as parenting classes and first aid training. For example, I would begin prenatal classes by asking participants what they already knew about human pregnancy and birth (present knowledge and previous experiences) and what they wanted to learn from the classes (immediate learning needs). Based on these needs and the content of the public health prenatal program, I would plan and deliver programs and invite participants to share their experiences. Often the experiences that people shared reinforced program content information. There was minimal mutual engagement.

Although adult learning practices in community health nursing were limited at this time, significant new thinking about the health care system was beginning to occur. There was a growing understanding that education of individuals was only one factor that could improve health. A key point in this movement was when Lalonde (1974) and the World Health Organization (WHO, 1978) identified other factors affecting health, both in the political context and in the socio-economic context. These factors are now referred to as the determinants of health (DOH) and the social determinants of health (SDOH). The work of identifying determinants of health (Evans, Barer, & Marmor, 1994) came to the forefront in the 1990s, clearly articulating the evidence of the many factors that contribute to ill health. Recent research supports the contextual factors affecting the health of people (WHO, 2003; WHO Commission on the Social Determinants of Health, 2008). This growing body of work had a direct effect on the practice of public health nursing, urging it to embrace community development and population-focused approaches that situated health within a myriad of factors beyond the individual. In the mid-'80s when Epp (1986) and the WHO (1986) introduced the Ottawa Charter for Health Promotion, there was a growing understanding that there are systemic issues implicit in health, such as access to services, programs, and education. The Ottawa Charter promoted at a universal level the value of health promotion. Although this charter had remnants of emphasis on disease prevention, it championed the need for a more collaborative approach to address health. This presaged the more intensive investigation of the determinants of health, the many different social and economic factors that affect health such as geography, income, education, and race. Based on the work of the Canadian Federal/Provincial/Territorial Advisory Committee on Population Health (1994) concerning the concept of determinants of health, Hamilton and Bhatti (1996) developed a population health framework and stressed the need for a health promotion approach that integrated an understanding of the determinants of health in a comprehensive strategy to improve the health of the population. Though terms such as 'health promotion' predominate, 'population health promotion' is often considered to be the more inclusive term.

Yet, the change from an individually focused and top-down model to a population-focused and community-centred model has not been complete. As a university teacher of community health nursing, my present challenge is to find strategies and projects in collaboration with nursing educators, community health colleagues, and community members to introduce nursing students to population-focused nursing practices. Many community nursing and public health nursing textbooks, both in discussions on health promotion and health education, continue to perpetuate a belief that 'adopting healthier behaviours or lifestyles is the key to health promotion' (Stamler & Yiu, 2005, p. 119). Even authors such as Edleman and Mandle (2006), who acknowledge the socio-political aspects of health and illness, still emphasize lifestyle changes. I struggle with the inadequacies in individual-focused nursing theory and health promotion models that do not stress the context – the determinants of health and inequities in health – and the real life context of the learning needs of populations.

To address the gap in the literature and in practice, I developed a Framework for Practice to direct my work and teaching in community health nursing. The Framework has grown from my experiences in public health nursing and adult education, and is routinely adjusted through praxis (Freire, 1970) – the interplay of action and reflection in undergraduate nursing education, community projects, and research. My discussion of the Framework (Table 10.1) is followed by examples of application by public health nurses and student nurses.

Framework for Population-Focused Nursing Practice

The three main components of my Framework are: (a) the knowledge fields of nursing, public health, and adult learning – each consists of theory, concepts, evidence, information, and principles associated with the fields; (b) the nursing process which consists of five steps – assessing, diagnosing, planning, implementing, evaluating (College of Registered Nurses of Nova Scotia (CRNNS), 2004, 2009; Community Health Nurses Association of Canada (CHNAC), 2003); and (c) integrative questions.

Table 10.1. A Framework for Population-Focused Nursing Practice

Theory	Process	Sample questions to integrate practice
Nursing theories/ models – for example, the community nursing process and the developmental stage of learners	ASSESSMENT	What do I know from theory that can be applied to my target population?
	NURSING DIAGNOSIS	Based on the assessment evidence, what are the key goals?
Health concepts – for example, functions of public health and determinants of health.	PLANNING	Are literacy/health literacy, cultural safety, and other ways of knowing taken into consideration?
	IMPLEMENTATION	Do teaching-learning methods relate to the learner and learning objectives?
		What is the evidence that goals were achieved?
Adult learning theory & concepts – for example, learning needs assessment and relating teaching-learning activities tools to learning goals.	EVALUATION	Were all elements of the Population Health Model covered?
		Are relationships established? Is there evidence of trust, collaboration, and participatory processes?

Using the nursing process as a guiding structure, and the three fields of knowledge as a frame of reference, I develop questions to guide the integration of the three fields as population-focused nursing practice. The Framework assists me in teaching-learning situations with nursing students, public health practitioners, and community members about a population-focused approach to public health.

Framework Component 1: Fields of Knowledge

Nursing. The first field of knowledge in my Framework is nursing theory and concepts that support nursing practice. Nursing theories generally focus on nurses 'doing' with/for clients, or motivating clients to learn and hence change behaviours to improve health outcomes. For instance, nursing in the community follows a community assessment process. The theory and the art of building a relationship with a population, a family, or a client is essential for public health nursing practice (Community Health Nurses Association of Canada (CHNAC), 2003; College of Registered Nurses of Nova Scotia (CRNNS), 2009). Stated by the CRNNS (2009) as the theoretical and practical knowledge of relational practice, the nursing profession acknowledges 'relational practice' and the 'nursing therapeutic relationship' as the foundation for all nursing practice (p. 24). My engagement with the field of adult learning expanded my knowledge and practice on how 'dialogue' can develop and build the relationship with groups, communities, and populations (Moseley, 2004).

Learning theories and models – developmental theories from Piaget and Erikson, the Stages of Change Model/Transtheoretical Model, Health Belief Model, Social Learning Theory, and Community Organization Theory (Murray, Zentner, Pangman, & Pangman, 2006; Potter, Perry, Ross-Kerr, & Wood, 2006; Stanhope, Lancaster, Jessup-Falcioni, & Viverais-Dresler, 2008) – can add some structure planning population health interventions depending on the population's identified needs. I also use the classic developmental theory (Edleman & Mandle, 2006), which focuses on individual growth and development at life stages; and the family theory (Friedman, Bowden, & Jones, 2008; Wright, & Leahey, 2009), which focuses on associated tasks of family members, both of which can be helpful in planning teaching-learning experiences for target groups.

When I apply these theories I am aware that many are focused on the individual and his/her lifestyle, and based on accepted Western culture. Hence they may not have validity for all groups in our communities; for example immigrants, First Nations peoples, and Inuit. I am inclined in this respect to also follow the work of the Aboriginal Learning Knowledge Centre (2007), of the Canadian Council on Learning, which has developed Holistic Lifelong Learning Models to recognize Indigenous ways of knowing.

Public Health. The second field of knowledge that I have built into my Framework is public health theory especially the Canadian Population Health Template (PHAC/Health Canada, 2001, 2008) for developing and evaluating health education and population health promotion projects and initiatives, and which is explicitly based on public health theory and sciences. Similar to the nursing process and community nursing, the Template follows a step-by-step process to analyse the health issue, set priorities, take action, and evaluate results. The Template identifies 'key elements' (Health Canada/PHAC, 2001) to meet its goals of increasing the health of the population and decreasing health status inequities. These key elements are: (a) measuring population health status; (b) analysing determinants of health; (c) basing decisions on evidence; (d) increasing 'upstream' interventions ('upstream' referring to policies and interventions that prevent sickness; (e) using multiple strategies; (f) involving the public; (g) collaborating across sectors; and, (h) being accountable for outcomes. I believe use of this Template in public health nursing builds evidence and helps increase knowledge (Arbuthnot, Hansen-Ketchum, Jewers, Moseley, & Wilson, 2007).

Although it is strong on theory, the Template (PHAC/Health Canada, 2001) does not clearly outline the 'how to' for relationship building. Yet, the Core Competencies for Public Health in Canada (PHAC, 2007a) acknowledge the importance of relationship competencies – skills, knowledge, and attitudinal values of public health: 'Important values in public health include a commitment to equity, social justice and sustainable development, recognition of the importance of health of the community as well as the individual, and respect for diversity, self-determination, empowerment and community participation' (p. 3). Clearly, another practical component is needed to build capacity among public health practitioners for dialogue and relationships.

In teaching I build on the science of public health. The science includes approaches and methods of epidemiology, demography, surveillance, natural history of disease, and levels of prevention. If a project focuses on a specific disease/condition in the population, then 'Measuring Population Health Status' from the Template (PHAC/Health Canada, 2001) can be used to frame the inclusion of incidence, prevalence, mortality rates for population groups and the natural history of the disease and/or the risk factors that predispose peoples to a condition/disease. The natural history of the disease/condition includes the stages of susceptibility, subclinical, clinical, and recovery, disability, or death. Applying levels of prevention to the stages of the natural history of the disease assists in planning interventions. The four levels of prevention include primordial (policy and legislation), primary (health promotion or specific protection such as immunization), secondary (screening and/or early detection of the condition/disease), and tertiary (support and rehabilitation). Primordial and primary prevention are interventions appropriate to the susceptibility stage, secondary prevention interventions are applicable to the subclinical stage, and tertiary prevention interventions are suitable for the stages of clinical and recovery/disability/death (Public Health Agency of Canada, 2007b). I emphasize that interventions can be planned for each of the levels of prevention. For example, we can apply this to cancer of the cervix in women. Recent studies link vaginal exposure to the infectious agent Human Papillomavirus (HPV) as part of the natural history of cancer of the cervix. Primordial and primary prevention interventions, focused at the susceptibility stage of the disease include policy to offer publicly funded HPV immunization to adolescents, social media marketing to educate the public, and provincial services to deliver the publicly funded immunization programs. Secondary prevention interventions include pap test screening for sexually active women, which is geared to detecting cervical dysplasia, precancerous cells, and cancer cells at the subclinical stage of the disease. Tertiary prevention interventions are aimed at cure and support of women with cervical cancer and include continuous follow-up and treatment protocols such as biopsy, hysterectomy, and radiation.

Adult learning. The third field of knowledge in my public health teaching Framework is adult learning. Writers such as Merriam, Caffarella, and Baumgartner (2007) agree that adult learning remains a form of social intervention, and that social interaction and dialogue shape the learning work just as much as the theory and research (p. 270). Merriam et al. build on Paulo Freire's 1970 work to support this view, especially on his notion that the authentic educational encounter is 'the process in which ... [we] achieve a deepening awareness both of the sociocultural reality which shapes their lives and of their capacity to transform that reality' (cited in Merriam et al., p. 262). From my perspective, the 'sociocultural reality' of people relates to the 'determinants of health' in the public health field. I believe adult education values coincide with the goals of public health, the 'why' of my Framework for Population-Focused Nursing Practice. Other important concepts and theories from adult education in my Framework support the 'how.' These include designing learning based on an understanding of the characteristics of adult learners and their varied learning styles, needs, and goals. The public health nurse as educator also needs to be skilled in creating learning objectives, employing learner-centred teaching-learning methods, and implementing effective evaluation techniques (Vella, 2002).

Key to effective learning, and integral to my Framework, is the principle of 'dialogue,' which is at the heart of effective adult learning principles (Vella, 2002). My scholarly engagement with the field of adult learning strengthened my knowledge and practice on how 'dialogue' builds the relationship and acknowledges the reality of the learner context (Moseley, 2004). Vella (2002) discusses 12 principles of effective adult education that she believes close the gap between teacher and learner to develop honest dialogue across cultures, sexes, classes, and ages (p.xiv). Central to this development of dialogue are principles such as needs assessment and safety. In using these, Vella is pointing to the importance of finding out informally and formally from participants what they need to learn, and to create an environment where it is safe to ask questions and to be critical of the learning process. For instance, in my practice as a public health nurse in Nova Scotia, school staff had identified issues among older teens of drug abuse, violence, low self-esteem, and unplanned pregnancy. In my needs assessment process, I sent a questionnaire to all students. They identified their first priority as issues around communication – with parents, boy/girlfriends, friends, and teachers. Together with a group of volunteer teens from the school drama club, we designed skits on communication that the students presented to all classes. Within the classes, confidentiality was required so that students felt safe to discuss whatever issue was most important to them.

Framework Component 2: The Nursing Process

The nursing process, Framework Component 2, gives structure to problem-solving in public health education. It 'is a systematic approach that applies knowledge from the biological, physical and social sciences ... to identify, diagnose, and treat human responses to health and illness' (Potter, Perry, Ross-Kerr, & Wood, 2006, p. 183). A nursing diagnosis is based on the analysis and interpretation of assessment data (CRNNS, 2009). A community assessment process follows the nursing process and includes public health sciences, building relationships with community, and developing programs to meet identified community needs (Vollman, Anderson, & McFarlane, 2004). I use the nursing process in my Framework to organize the guiding questions to follow a problem-solving model. Following the five steps in the nursing process helps me to identify the source of information/evidence from each of the three fields in order to answer the guiding questions.

Framework Component 3: Questions to Integrate Practice

The third Framework Component, questions to integrate practice, is the place in my Framework where I bring together the bodies of knowledge of nursing, public health, and adult learning by challenging students with questions. The questions guide the process of identifying and applying information from the fields of knowledge to a specific issue with a group or population. Questions are framed within the nursing process to support a population-focused nursing approach that is 'relational.' The questions also support the idea of applying theory and evidence to practice, in order to know the 'why' and 'how' of evidenced-informed practice. For example, theory of community development includes community involvement in all aspects of the process to identify and take action on issues affecting the health of a community (Stanhope et al., 2008). Capacity-building action includes assessing community assets, recognizing strengths, and mobilizing community partners; this is a Community Health Nursing Standard of Practice (CHNAC, 2003).

Application of the Framework

One example from my teaching practice where I apply this Framework is in a collaborative partnership with local public health nurses, high schools, and student nurses. For six years the partnership provided opportunities for second-year nursing students to apply content and theory, which they studied in a population-focused community health nursing course. I use the Framework for Population-Focused Nursing practice to guide the experience of working with a group of student nurses to offer a public health project on sexual health in local high schools.

Assessment

After discussion with the school's public health nurse, principle, and guidance counsellors, we obtain permission to implement a project. We begin our planning of a sexual health education project for adolescents by thinking about the related developmental theory that can be connected to capacities for learning about sexuality and sexual health. For example, knowledge of Piaget's cognitive stage, Formal Concrete Operational, assists us to understand that this age group is acquiring the ability to think systematically about all logical relations within a problem, and that they are interested in abstract ideas and the process of thinking (Murray et al., 2006). According to the psychosocial development theory of Erikson, most adolescents are working to achieve a sense of personal identity by separating from family and searching for their beliefs, which affects their motivation and readiness to learn (Potter & Perry, 2006). Review of relevant theory includes knowledge of human growth and development, which situates puberty and body changes within this age group, so we imagine that planning topics might include menstruation, fertility, harm reduction practices, emotional changes, and gender identification, to name a few. Another question we often have at the assessment stage is: What do we know about this specific, regional, and local group of teens? A literature review yields regional and provincial reports and consultations, as well as research on adolescent sexuality, health statistics on STIs, adolescent pregnancy incidence, and other data on conditions of concern. The school public health nurse validates incident rates locally. A further source of information for our educational sessions comes from the provincial Department of Education curriculum that outlines content on sexual health for the school grade.

We are then challenged to ask what we know about the condition/disease and what determinants of health affect health conditions in this population. Statistics Canada provides us with demographics for the region; as well, the District Health Authority and Public Health Services health assessment assists us in identifying determinants of health affecting the sexual health of the adolescent population: culture, social norms, accessibility of health services, condoms, and so on. Analysis of determinants of health for our locale includes the fact that we may be working with a rural population, with limited access to services (e.g., birth control, pregnancy tests, condoms), low socio-economic status, Scottish culture, conservative social norms, and predominantly Roman Catholic religious beliefs. Statistics on communicable disease (STIs) show high incidence of Chlamydia for Nova Scotia. Patho-physiology information gives us the 'natural history' of common STIs. Knowledge of levels of prevention provides students and public health nurses with the process of identifying what key information this population group may need.

We then move to identifying stakeholders and finding out how we can build a relationship with them. In this case, a student committee, with the public health nurse as a member, was actively involved in requesting the sexual health presentations in one school. They validated key topics and wanted yearly sessions for all students in grades 8 to12, with information prepared to answer student-identified questions. We indicated we were willing to respond to the challenge.

Adult learning came into play next. We asked: What are important adult education principles and concepts? How can we honour and respect the target population's learning needs? What is the learner's context? Based on our review of the literature, curriculum, and research, we developed a needs assessment questionnaire and gave it to the high school students. Results of the pre-session questionnaire showed readiness to learn, previous knowledge, and experiences.

Diagnosis/Priorities

Based on the assessment evidence, the next questions we asked were: What are the key goals? Have the priorities and goals been validated by the target group, community, and population? Do these priorities relate to public health functions? Based on a discussion with stakeholders, and a review of education curriculum, research, and reports, as well as the needs assessment questionnaire, we came to see that the priority topics were healthy relationships, sexuality, STI's, pap smear screening, breast health, and testicular self exam. These topics relate to the public health functions of Health Promotion, Disease and Injury Prevention.

Planning. Once the diagnosis was complete, we moved to planning. Using the key goals that we had identified, we began planning each topic presentation using adult learning concepts to write objectives. We were concerned about respecting the learners' needs for safety and confidentiality as well as to encourage active participation in learning, so we deliberately designed engagement methods of return demonstrations and role playing. We used specific learning activities from the Canadian Guidelines on Sexual Health Education (PHAC, 2008b), which support active learning. One of our questions related to how we might use the Population Health Promotion Template to assist with planning and evaluating interventions. We located measures of health status for the population group in this region and compared these to provincial and national statistics, with the intent of sharing this information with the high school students: for example, information on incidence of STI statistics and adolescent pregnancies. Along with identifying this information, we used a number of other strategies, such as making sure the public health nurse was accessible to high school students for follow-up; having the principal obtain the school board's permission; asking the school guidance and public health officials for specific information resources; ensuring that the university School of Nursing had breast and testicular models we could use; making sure that the topics we identified also followed the approved education curriculum; and notifying parents for permission and also inviting them to attend an information session.

We planned the sexual health presentations to meet needs identified by the adolescents on the topics they had identified, such as 'healthy relationships' and testicular self-examination. The nursing students prepared lesson plans that addressed the developmental stage of the learner, needs assessment data, learner objectives, adult learning strategies and methods, and audiovisual aids, as well as the need to set evaluation criteria to measure learning objectives. The nursing students prepared posters and other visual aids, and the public health nurses prepared a resource handout. Care was taken to ensure that literacy and health literacy were taken into consideration, especially if the student needs assessment questionnaire raised literacy issues. The nursing students prepared topics on healthy sexuality for presentations of eight to 10 minutes, to rotating small groups of five to 12 adolescents.

Implementation. As we began to implement the sessions, we kept asking: How can the interventions be respectful and engage the young people in a meaningful way? We utilized guides for best practices for adolescent teaching-learning, such as the Canadian Guidelines on Sexual Health Education (CPHA, 2008b), since we were aware that active learning was important in order to engage adolescents. We implemented a presentation on 'healthy relationships' by following the Experiential Learning Cycle (Cameron, 1999); a scenario was role played by the nursing students, then learners were asked to reflect on the scenario, identify if it contained a positive or negative relationship, and why. The high school students were asked to discuss their own values; identify assertive verbal responses they might apply for future situations; and discuss risks factors such as peer pressure, low self-esteem, drugs, and alcohol, which might affect decisions. We closed by asking for volunteers to demonstrate the scenario. In all sessions, the nursing student utilized his/her knowledge of the relational practice to develop a safe and trusting dialogue with the high school students. Nursing students had been coached in how to handle difficult questions and behaviours respectfully and professionally, and this came through in their actual delivery. The high school students demonstrated engagement by participating in interactive activities, which included return demonstrations of condom application, use of breast and testicular models to discover 'lumps and bumps,' and asking questions.

Evaluation. In the last phase we asked: What is the evidence that goals were achieved? Was learning transferred and did the new learning have an impact on the population, on key stakeholders, and on the high school students? We were most curious about whether we could evaluate the impact over the long term, for example was there a change in health status data. Other questions included: Was evaluation information given back to the population? Were all elements of the Population Health Template covered? To answer some of these questions, we gave a post-session questionnaire to the high school students, teachers, guidance counsellors, and public health nurses. Participants were asked for feedback to improve format, content, and methods. A summary of evaluation data was sent to the participants. The data showed evidence of benefits to both adolescents and nursing students, which the collaborating partners continue to refer to as a 'win-win' experience.

Summary

The guiding questions follow the nursing process to facilitate application of knowledge and theory to practice, and to facilitate the integration of the three fields of knowledge: nursing, public health, and adult learning. This integration permitted a comprehensive population-focused approach for public health practice that each field could not deliver alone. Adult learning principles and practices contributed the 'how to' of relational practice and dialogue useful in connecting with people within populations. It was my observation that professional relationships and connections were vital to fulfil the need for public participation in this health education process. The foundation standards of public health nurses supported relational practice (i.e., the 'why'), and adult education principles specified the 'how' to establish relationships and effective participation of the population. Honouring the lived experiences of learners was brought in through our use of adult education principles. It was my observation that in all population-focused health initiatives and health promotion endeavours, the living context and experience of the population need as much weight as public health science. In fact, health information and knowledge transfer to the population and public is often rhetorical if adult education principles and concepts are not applied.

The Framework's questions allowed me to integrate three knowledge fields – nursing, public health, and adult learning – the basics of population-focused nursing practice. In our commitment to integrate adult learning throughout the Framework we were called to be account-able to, respect, and focus on the learners in the health educational pro-cess. Adult learning supported relational practice and challenged us to respect the unique context in which we were working, so that we avoided delivering a program that was top down and in which the health profes-sionals were set up as 'experts.'

Use of the Framework demonstrates that it can assist public health nurses to shift the perspective in health promotion from the individual medical model to the system view of population health. The strength of the population health view is that it assesses the context of the pop-ulation (e.g., health status, determinants of health) and evaluates the outcomes. For example, linking health status measurement with evalu-ation of services and programs can identify inequities in health among populations. Knowledge of context, as identified by the population, is essential to achieve public health goals of protecting, promoting, and restoring the health of all the people through collective or social actions, and to reduce inequities of health in our Canadian population. This is a concern of many of the writers in this collection, including Ronson and Irving, as well as Egan, and Chovanec and Johnson.

Use of the Framework for Population-focused Nursing Practice reminds me that I am only one part of a whole. From my perspective, this is a proper return to the roots of Canadian Medicare, where a health pro-fessional brings knowledge and evidence from her/his field, and the population brings knowledge of context, to make decisions and learn together as partners, resulting in democracy in health.

REFERENCES

Arbuthnot, E., Hansen-Ketchum, P.A., Jewers, H., Moseley, J., & Wilson, C. (2007). Bringing theory to life: Engaging students in a collaborative population-based screening project. International Journal of Nursing Education Scholarship, 11(4), 191–196.

Canadian Council on Learning, Aboriginal Learning Knowledge Centre. (2007). Redefining how success is measured in First Nations, Inuit and Métis learning. Retrieved 16 February 2010 from http://cli.ccl-cca.ca/FN/index.php?q=home.

Cameron, B. (1999). Active learning: Green guide #2. The Society for Teaching and Learning in Higher Education. London, ON: University of Western Ontario Bookstore. www.stlhe.ca/en/publications/green_guides/index.php.

College of Registered Nurses of Nova Scotia. (2004). Standards for nursing practice. Halifax: Author. Retrieved 16 February 2010 from http://www.crnns.ca/documents/standards2004.pdf.

College of Registered Nurses of Nova Scotia. (2009). Entry-level competencies for registered nurses in Nova Scotia. Halifax: Author. Retrieved 16 February 2010 from http://www.crnns.ca/documents/Entry-Level_Competencies2009.pdf.

Community Health Nurses Association of Canada. (2003). Canadian Community Health Nursing Standards of Practice. Retrieved 17 May 2010 from http://www.chnc.ca/nursing-standards-of-practice.cfm.

Edleman, C.L., & Mandle, C.L. (2006). Health promotion throughout the life span. (6th ed.). St. Louis, MO: Mosby.

Epp, J. (1986). Achieving health for all: A framework for health promotion. Ottawa: Minister of Supply and Services Canada, Health and Welfare Canada. Retrieved 17 may 2010 from http://www.bvsde.paho.org/bvsacd/cd68/paho557/s5.pdf.

Evans, R.G., Barer, M.L., & Marmor, T.R. (1994). Why are some people healthy and others not? New York: Aldine de Gruyter.

Federal/Provincial/Territorial Advisory Committee on Population Health. (1994). Strategies for population health: Investing in the health of Canadians. Ottawa: Health and Welfare Canada. Retrieved 17 May 17 2010 from http://www.phac-aspc.gc.ca/ph-sp/pdf/strateg-eng.pdf.

Freire, P. (1970). Pedagogy of the oppressed. New York: Continuum.

Friedman, M., Bowden, V.R., & Jones, E.G. (2008). Family nursing: Research, theory and practice (5th ed.). Norwalk, NJ: Appleton & Lange.

Hamilton, N., & Bhatti, T. (1996). An integrated model of population health and health promotion: A working draft. Ottawa: Health Promotion Development Division, Government of Canada.

Lalonde, M. (1974). A new perspective on the health of Canadians. Retrieved 16 May from http://198.103.98.171/ph-sp/pdf/perspect-eng.pdf.

Last, J.M. (Ed.). (2001). A dictionary of epidemiology (4th ed.). New York: Oxford Press.

Merriam, S.B., Caffarella, R.S., & Baumgartner, L.M. (2007). Learning in adulthood: A comprehensive guide (3d ed.). San Francisco: Jossey-Bass.

Moseley, J. (2004). Using appreciative inquiry to evaluate the teaching-learning process of senior community nursing students. St Francis Xavier University: Author. Unpublished Masters in Adult Education thesis.

Murray, R.B., Zentner, J.P., Pangman, V., & Pangman, C. (2006). Health promotion strategies through the lifespan. Toronto: Pearson.

National Advisory Committee on SARS and Public Health. (2003). Learning from SARS: Renewal of public health in Canada. Ottawa: Heath Canada.

Potter, P.A., Perry, A.G., Ross-Kerr, J.C., & Wood, M.J. (2006). Canadian fundamentals of nursing (3d ed.). St. Louis, MO: Elsevier Mosby.

Public Health Agency of Canada/Health Canada. (2001). The Population Health Template Working Tool. Ottawa: Government of Canada. Retrieved 17 May 2010 from http://www.phac-aspc.gc.ca/ph-sp/pdf/template_tool-eng.pdf.

Public Health Agency of Canada. (2007). Core competencies for public health in Canada. Retrieved 20 April 2009 from http://www.phac-aspc.gc.ca/ccph-cesp/index-eng.php.

Public Health Agency of Canada. (2008a). Population Health Approaches: An Organizing Framework. Retrieved 3 December 2009 from http://cbpp-pcpe.phac-aspc.gc.ca/population_health/index-eng.html.

Public Health Agency of Canada. (2008b). Canadian guidelines on sexual health (Rev. ed.). Ottawa: Author. Retrieved 16 May 2010 from http://198.103.98.171/publicat/cgshe-ldnemss/pdf/guidelines-eng.pdf.

Shah, C. (2003). Public health and preventive medicine in Canada (5th ed.). Toronto: Elsevier Canada.

Stamler, L.L., & Yiu, L. (2005). Community health nursing: A Canadian perspective. Toronto: Pearson/Prentice Hall.

Stanhope, M., Lancaster, J., Jessup-Falcioni, H., & Viverais-Dresler, G.A. (2008). Community health nursing in Canada (1st Canadian ed.). Toronto: Mosby/Elsevier.

Vella, J. (2002). Learning to listen: Learning to teach (Rev. ed.). San Francisco: Jossey-Bass.

Vollman, A.R., Anderson, E.T., & McFarlane, J. (2004). Canadian community as partner. Philadelphia: Lippincott.

World Health Organization. (1978). Declaration of Alma-Alta. Retrieved 17 May 2010 from http://www.who.int/hpr/NPH/docs/declaration_almaata.pdf.

World Health Organization. (1986). Ottawa charter for health promotion: Health for all by the year 2000. Retrieved 17 May 2010 from http://www. who.int/hpr/NPH/docs/ottawa_charter_hp.pdf.

World Health Organization Centre for Urban Health. (2003). Social deter- minants of health: The solid facts. Ed. Richard Wilkinson and Michael Marmot. Copenhagen, Denmark: Centre for Urban Health, World Health Organization. Retrieved 17 May 2010 from http://www.euro.who.int/docu ment/e81384.pdf.

World Health Organization's Commission on the Social Determinants. (2008). Closing the gap in a generation: Health equity through action on the social determinants of health. Geneva & Denmark: WHO Press. Retrieved 17 May 2010 from http://whqlibdoc.who.int/publications/2008/9789241563703_ eng.pdf.

Wright, L.M., & Leahey, M. (2009). Nurses and families: A guide to family assessment and intervention (5th ed.). Philadelphia: F.A Davis.

11 Beyond Healthy Aging: The Practice of Narrative Care in Gerontology

BILL RANDALL

> Every time an old person dies, it's like a library burns down.
>
> – Alex Haley

Recently, my 90-year-old father suffered a spell of dizziness and weakness that made us fearful he was having a stroke. We dialled 911 and rushed him to the emergency room. Fortunately, his ECG and bloodwork checked out normal for his age, and in less than two hours he was free to return home. Before we left, however, a kindly nurse approached us and explained that her role was to advocate for patients over 65. Among other things, this meant determining what their needs might be by way of grab bars, mobility aids, and the like, which, if met, could keep them that much longer in their homes. She informed us of various assessments that could be done, and even offered to contact the Department of Social Services on our behalf. As a gerontologist, what struck me most about her, though, was her skill in putting my father at ease, how she looked straight at him, and spoke so that he could hear her, yet in no way talked down to him. Above all, it was her implicit sensitivity to him, not as a 'patient' or a 'case,' but as a person, with a lifetime of experiences and stories behind him. By her very manner, she was embodying *narrative care*.

Narrative care is core care, a fundamental element in attending to another person's needs. And it ought to run through everything we do within the health care field – especially where older adults are involved (Bohlmeijer, Kenyon, & Randall, 2011). In what follows, I will be drawing on recent thinking in '*narrative* gerontology' to sketch what such care entails and how we can learn to practise it more effectively, whatever the role we hold, or are preparing to hold: for example, doctor, nurse, social worker, chaplain, physiotherapist, psychotherapist, or director of recreation – to name but a few. But before I proceed, I need to talk about 'autobiographical learning,' something which later life particularly, I believe, invites us to pursue. And to set things up to talk about that, I need to say a word about narrative gerontology itself, beginning with what I fear goes missing in campaigns aimed at 'healthy aging.'

Healthy Aging, Successful Aging, and Mental Fitness

The increasing emphasis on healthy aging is, no doubt, essential. Overeating, under-exercising, too much salt or sugar in our diets, too much alcohol or tobacco – these can take a major toll on elders' lives, in the form, say, of heart disease or diabetes; of trips to the doctor and reliance on medication; and, in general, of diminished quality of life. And this says nothing of the cost to the health care system as a whole. Concepts of healthy aging are variations on 'successful aging' (Rowe & Kahn, 1998). Successful aging concerns three key components of our lives: the physical, the social, and the cognitive. Accordingly, the 'successful' older person is the one who keeps in good physical condition, stays involved with family and community, and remains cognitively and mentally alert. The concept gained attention in the 1990s as a reaction to stereotypes of later life as a period of inevitable deterioration. Yet, inspiring as it is, the successful aging paradigm can be critiqued from various angles (Holstein & Minkler, 2003). For one, it is tacitly elitist, in that only those who manage to stay healthy and engaged are by definition successful. It also sidesteps the fact that, technically, all of us *fail* at aging, since sooner or later we die. And borrowing from gerontologist Gene Cohen (2005), the notion of successful aging 'presents the goal as minimizing decline rather than recognizing the huge potential for positive growth in later life' (p. xxiif). Albeit implicitly, successful aging frames aging per se in terms of a 'narrative of decline' (Gullette, 1997).

In gerontology in general and geriatrics in particular, it is this 'huge potential for positive growth' that often goes unacknowledged. Even in *educational* gerontology, our understanding of 'learning' in later life tends towards the functional. It concerns learning how to *do* things, or learning *about* things, or maintaining 'mental fitness' (Cusack & Thompson, 2003) through doing quizzes, crosswords, puzzles, and the like. All of this is well and good. But in the process, a deeper, more soulful type of learning – learning about oneself, that is – gets quietly eclipsed, and, with it, a more optimistic perspective on aging itself. For beneath the emphasis on mental fitness lurks the sense that, in the end, the most we can hope for is to delay our inevitable decline. And beneath that again lies the perception of aging as a disease, as something we can die of. In short, aging is medicalized, pathologized – as all too often are the elderly themselves. Though the aim of 'healthy aging' is admirable, then, it fails to go far enough, for it downplays our potential for 'aging in-depth' (Bianchi, 1991, p. 60). Such aging, I suggest, is associated with *autobiographical* learning, a mode of learning which health care workers themselves can play a vital role in encouraging. But, first, let me distinguish between two broad ways of understanding 'aging': outside versus inside.

Outside Aging versus Inside Aging

Aging on the outside, as it were, is biological aging or physical aging. It is what happens to our bodies and our brains. In this respect, the narrative of decline is rooted in reality, for the news is not exactly good: hair falling out (or coming in) where we wish it would not, loss of bone mass and muscle tone, slowing of reaction time, plus the numerous conditions to which such changes make us vulnerable. Happily, this is not the whole story of aging. Aging on the inside, as it were, is what happens in our minds (versus our brains) and in our understanding of who we are. It is what happens in our experience of ourselves through time. We can call this *biographical* aging (Ruth & Kenyon, 1996), or simply psychological aging. Naturally, outside and inside, biological and biographical, physical and psychological, are tightly entwined. Witness the oft-noted link between *psyche* and *soma,* a link we note with added urgency in the case of dementia, where changes in the brain seem tied to changes in personality. But the biographical side of aging, which is every bit as intricate and important as the biological side, has been vastly understudied. Even in the psychology of aging, certainly where the topic of memory is concerned, the focus remains far more on the *mechanics* of memory (e.g., on deficits in encoding information, in speed of retrieval and accuracy of recall) than on the *meanings* our memories may possess for us, and on how those meanings can evolve over time.

Put simply, then, biological-physical-outside aging is about deterioration and decline. Biographical-psychological-inside aging, however, can involve continuing development – development in self-understanding, development in wisdom – development which age itself in no way needs to limit. It can involve (actively, consciously) *growing* old and not just (passively, inexorably) *getting* old. And key to growing old, whatever else it may entail, is what adult educator Wilhelm Mader (1995) calls 'biographical self-reflection,' something he says 'no educational material, no subject matter' cannot "trigger"' (p. 245). Indeed, triggering it, one can argue, should be our overarching aim. As fellow educator Michael Brady (1990) asks, 'Is this not our destiny as human beings, to learn, to grow, to come to know ourselves and the meanings of our life in the deepest, most textured way possible? If we do not know the self, what can we know?' (p. 51).

Narrative Gerontology and the Storied Nature of Identity

Biographical aging is a central focus of 'narrative gerontology' (Kenyon, Clark, & de Vries, 2001; Kenyon, Bohlmeijer, & Randall, 2011), a core premise of which is that human beings are not just physical beings or medical beings but interpretive beings, meaning-making beings. Aided by our capacity for language, it is this, in fact, that most distinguishes us from other forms of life. We are 'the story species' (Gold, 2002), insofar as the primary way we make sense of what happens in our lives – in sickness and in health alike – is through narrative. It is through weaving and reweaving, telling and retelling, what, in the end, are *stories* – big and little, long and short, true and not so true, about the past and the future both. It is in terms of these stories that we identify our 'self,' that we believe and feel, act and think. Indeed, as a growing number of researchers are confirming, our propensity for making stories is wired into our brains (Fireman, McVay, & Flanagan, 2003). The narrative impulse has neurological roots – one more way the biological and biographical are married.

While this impulse is one we carry with us from an early age, its expression is integral to the development of identity in adolescence, when we awaken in earnest to our 'biographicity' (Alheit, 1995, p. 65), and certainly in mid- and later life as well (McAdams, 1996). Indeed, later life presents us with unique developmental tasks, whether or not we undertake them consciously. Pivotal among them is looking back upon our life, and, ideally, arriving at a sense of satisfaction with how it has unfolded and who we have become along the way. Indeed, the urge to engage in *life review* has been identified as an essential, if not universal, experience as we age (Butler, 2007). Carrying it out immerses us in a process that is potentially transformative in nature. It is a *narrative* process, too, because what we look back upon are, in the end, our memories. And our memories – autobiographical memories, that is – are narrative constructions (Rubin, 1995, p. 2). They are not just straight recordings of what took place; they are edited interpretations, storied reproductions, odd blends of fact and fictionalization that could more fairly be called *factions*. Memory, if you will, is a matter of faction – an insight that becomes easier to accept once we realize that what we remember is ever but a fraction of what we have experienced. When we think back over our life, in other words, what we think back over is not our life itself, in all its raw detail. It is not the *history* of our life, so much as the *story* of our life – or, more accurately, the *stories* in terms of which we understand that life. Yet these stories are central to our identity, to who we are (Randall, 1995) – a point it is critical to bear in mind if we seek to relate insightfully to the people in our care.

Autobiographical Learning, Later Life, and Narrative Foreclosure

Autobiographical learning, I am proposing, is learning about ourselves and from ourselves through the stories by which we define our *selves* (see also Nelson, 1994). And it can take a variety of forms: guided autobiography (Birren & Deutchman, 1991), dynamic reminiscence (Chandler & Ray, 2002), creative reminiscence (Bohlmeijer, Valenkamp, Westerhof, Smit, & Cuijpers, 2005), life-story writing (Ray, 2000), or storytelling activities of several sorts, among them psychotherapy, which is nothing if not a narrative endeavour (McLeod, 1997). At its heart, however, autobiographical learning involves not just *telling* our stories, as healing as that can be. It is learning 'to listen to what our stories tell us' (Hampl, 1999, p. 33). Indeed, certain of our stories may have more to tell us than others. Many we have told over and over, to different audiences for differing reasons: to elicit a given reaction (e.g., laughter, pity, respect) or to communicate something about ourselves that, at bottom, we want our audience to know. And some of these, in turn, are ones we tell because they centre on events that are especially 'self-defining' (Singer & Blagov, 2004). Examples would be the stories that cluster around the period between, say, 15 and 30 when several huge changes are apt to be happening in our lives: pursuing an education, landing a career, finding a partner, beginning a family of our own. Depicted on a graph, such stories form the so-called 'reminiscence bump' (Neisser & Libby, 2000, p. 318). We recite these stories fairly often (if only to ourselves) because they concern memories that have extra meaning for us, because something in them begs to be reflected on, examined. Examining our stories – or 'reading our lives' (Randall & McKim, 2008) – is the heart of autobiographical learning, perhaps *the* learning that later life permits us. Moreover, certain age-related changes may make such learning easier, not harder, for us to do.

With retirement, or with the children at last on their own, later life affords many of us a marked increase in disposable time. While this can open the door to boredom or to a sense of having no purpose, it provides us greater opportunity to tackle the developmental work that I noted above: the 'philosophic homework' (Schacter-Shalomi & Miller, 1995, pp. 124–126) of sorting out our life thus far, and (so to speak) preparing for its final chapters – ideally, chapters characterized not by depression and despair but by meaning and fulfilment. It opens up a time in which time itself is experienced in different ways (see McFadden & Atchley, 2001). Our sense of the future, for example, shifts quietly within our consciousness and assumes a different *feel*. Similarly, our sense of the past can change as well, inasmuch as time-gone-by grows thicker and more compelling than time-to-come. Along with a different experience of personal time can also come a change in our experience of social space. In pulling back from the workaday world and the duties that structured our lives while raising our family or pursuing a career, we can undergo a degree of disengagement. This alone can issue in a changed relationship to our self and our story both. Then there are changes in the brain itself.

Gerontologist Gene Cohen (2005), whose thinking expands on notions of 'mental fitness,' undermines perceptions of aging as inevitable decline. Citing evidence from neuroscience, he argues that 'the brain is far more flexible and adaptable than once thought. Not only does [it] retain its capacity to form new memories, which entails making new connections between brain cells, but it can grow entirely new brain cells.' Moreover, 'older brains can process information in a dramatically different way than younger brains' (p. xv) – what psychologists call 'postformal thought' (Labouvie-Vief, 2000). Especially relevant here is what Cohen (2005) says about the 'Inner Push' (p. 31) towards 'autobiographical expression' (p. 22): 'Autobiographical writing and storytelling among older adults is common, and it stems from a variety of impulses, some psychological...and some physical. Autobiographical expression in the second half of life...is related to a rearrangement of brain functions that makes it easier to merge the speech, language, and sequential thinking typical of the left hemisphere with the creative, synthesizing right hemisphere' (pp. 22–23).

Obviously, Cohen is referring to the potential inherent in so-called *normal* aging. Dementia would appear to be another story (Randall, 2010). Yet people afflicted with dementia, it can be argued, are nonetheless persons with stories, even if their capacity to articulate those stories is different from our own. They can still be biographically active, still narratively developing, in ways we are not yet able to appreciate (Crisp, 1995). Moreover, behind their puzzling behaviours and odd confabulations can run storylines which, once we have some sense of them, place things in perspective. In addition, dementia draws attention to what, from a narrative perspective, is a pivotal theme: we do not story our lives in an existential vacuum but, directly or not, within complex webs of personal relationships (with parents, partners, peers) and narrative environments (of families, communities, churches, cultures). Narratively speaking, our lives are interwoven. Story-wise, no one is an island. Tragic as it is, therefore, dementia merely reminds us of this fundamental truth. It invites us – as family members, staff, and so on – to embrace our role as co-authors and keepers of the dementing person's story, as makers of meaning on their behalf. It invites us to keep the story open *for* them. This suggests the possibility of something even more tragic than dementia, something to which many can succumb: narrative foreclosure.

Narrative foreclosure, proposes psychologist Mark Freeman (2010), is 'the conviction that the story of one's life has effectively ended' (p. 125). Clearly, we can be gripped by such a conviction at any stage – the statistics on teen suicide serving as stark reminders. Still, later life itself presents conditions that make narrative foreclosure an obvious option. The same changes in time and space that invite us to engage in 'conscious aging' (Randall & Kenyon, 2001) can seed in us the sense that our life might just as well be finished, that little more of meaning lies ahead. Add to this a condition like arthritis or diabetes, or a terminal diagnosis, plus perhaps a lifelong awkwardness with looking inward anyway, and it is easy to understand how the elderly are vulnerable to 'arrested aging' (McCullough, 1993) – above all, when the prevailing narrative of aging per se is one of decline. 'Is this what my life has come to? Will this be my story from now on out – a story of pain, of loneliness, of death?' This sense of having to give in to one's narrative fate, so to speak, lies at the heart of our challenge when working with older patients. How do we help them keep their stories open? How do we help them sustain a good, strong story to counter the restrictions that sickness can impose upon their sense of self? Meeting this challenge means learning the practice of narrative care.

The Practice of Narrative Care

On the one hand, then, we have the inner push towards autobiographical expression, towards autobiographical learning and continuing narrative development – things that the conditions and transitions of later life (including illness) invite us to undertake. On the other hand, we have the pull to narrative foreclosure. The question is: What can we do as health care professionals to help ensure that push triumphs over pull? How can we assist our older patients-persons in growing old and not just getting old? Before going further, though, we need to be realistic.

Whatever the context (e.g., acute care, long-term care), health care is busy, stressful work. Given ever-shrinking budgets, persuading administrators to free up funds to set up programs of narrative care could seem futile from the start. But here is the point: narrative care is not some esoteric frill to be added onto everything else, if time allows. It is core care (Bohlmeijer, Kenyon, & Randall, 2011). By the same token, it need not be *costly* care. Compared with complex procedures and hi-tech equipment, it is remarkably cheap. It might actually *save* money, in fact, by reducing the incidence of 'problem behaviours' or the need for medications, and, most importantly, by enhancing patient self-esteem. Ultimately, it is not about quantity of time (and therefore money) but about quality of connection. It is not about how long we spend with particular patients or the techniques we may employ, so much as how well we *listen*. It is thus about gradually transforming the environments in which we work by honouring the centrality of stories, both our patients' and our own. This emphasis on story and the centrality of working with experience runs through many of the chapters in this book – Brookfield; Coady and Cameron; and Chovanec and Johnson, to name a few.

Our Patients' Stories. Advances in the realm of 'narrative medicine' are inspiring health care professionals to acknowledge the intimate bond between the stories patients tell about their lives and the symptoms and conditions they experience (Charon, 2006). They are inviting nurses and doctors to develop a more nuanced appreciation for the intricacy of their patients' worlds by exposing them to works of narrative art – novels, for example – that mediate in-depth insights into the experience of being and becoming 'a patient.' In short, it is urging them to listen more attentively to the stories of the persons they strive to help. Such listening, I propose, involves listening *to,* listening *for,* and listening *behind.*

Once more, of course, much of the listening that happens in health care contexts has to happen while carrying out our other duties – except perhaps in *palliative* care, where added time is presumably allotted to be present with the dying patient. But most medical settings are incredibly hectic, so we must learn to listen in strategic ways. Also, much of what a patient says to us will, understandably, concern the pain they are experiencing or the operation they are dreading. Yet as occasions arise – sooner rather than later, ideally; on admission to their room, for instance – we might say: 'I have a few minutes before I have to go. I'd like to learn a little more about you. Can you tell me a bit about yourself?' Such 'biographical encounters' (Kenyon & Randall, 1997, p. 144) can consume mere minutes of our time, but amid them we can gain rich (if broad brush) pictures of the persons for whom we are care: *I grew up on a farm, got married at 20, moved here with my husband, and was a housewife all my life. But I've always loved to garden. I remember this one time when. . . .* And then they might recount some anecdote that they have trotted out many times before, because, through it, they can introduce themselves to us, granting us a glimpse into their inner world and affording us a sense not so much of their medical *history* as of their personal *story*.

First, then, it is critical to listen to the *content* of their story; to the what, who, where, and when. If we have ears to hear, we can glean considerable information in a short span of time, not just *factual* information but *contextual* information: their life-situation, their background, culture, hobbies, and beliefs; the stress they may feel (and the internal stories that feed it), and the metaphors by which they define themselves – self-as-loser, -martyr, -hero, and so on. Much of this information, if properly charted, could prove valuable later on; for example, when deciding which treatment to pursue or when dealing with members of their family. But such listening should not be driven by an instrumental agenda alone. It is about getting a tentative sense of what it is like to *be* them – tentative, because subsequent encounters could require revising initial impressions. It is about developing empathy as much as acquiring information. It is learning about the patient as a *person*.

Listening *for* means listening for the *how* of *what* they say, for the 'storying style' to which they default (Randall, 1995, pp. 308–328), for any telltale postures or gestures, any shrugging of shoulders or furrowing of brows. Listening *for* means being attentive to verbal language and body language both, and to possible discrepancies between them. And it means being attentive to how the patient's story sparks reactions that arise from unresolved issues in our own story, reactions we do well to note yet not let them distract us.

Listening for also means listening for the back stories and the larger stories, the master narratives, that lie behind the what and the how alike: stories that offer us clues about the *why*. Listening *behind,* as I call it, means listening between the lines for the stories they are not telling us, but could if they knew us better: the abusive family; the neighbourhood they grew up in; the creed subscribed to; the secrets and convictions that give context to their attitudes and actions in the present. It means 'hearing *into* the narrative' (Kennedy, 1976, p. 108). It means asking ourselves why this version of their life and not some other, and what version they might wish to tell instead? Above all, attentive listening requires attentiveness, not slouching or yawning or darting glances at our pagers, not interrupting with 'uh-huh' or 'yeah' or other sounds that can signal we are not really listening at all, but simply impatient with the pace of their telling. It means conveying the impression that they are not just another patient but a unique individual with a unique story that extends beyond their circumstances here and now, of lying in an unfamiliar bed with uniformed professionals coming and going in a room they share with a stranger.

Listening to, for, and behind means being alert to narrative foreclosure as well; to signs, for instance, that their present situation of waiting for the test results, the surgery, the pain to resume, has become their *whole* story, instead of one more chapter, however bleak, in a story that has had other chapters before it and will have others to come. Listening in such ways means being alert to little opportunities to help them restory their current circumstances such that their identity does not revolve entirely around their illness – such that *having* cancer is not also *being* cancer. But it does not mean just cheering them up: 'Oh, you'll feel better tomorrow, dear!' It means being alert to opportunities to help open their story out from the cramped version they feel it reduced to in the present. This is no small matter, for in those delicate occasions when we take a minute here or there to listen to them as well as we can, a difference can be made. The person will feel that much more respected and appreciated, more deeply themselves. Surely, this can only aid the healing process. Author Henri Nouwen (1976), writing on the theme of 'hospitality,' puts the matter beautifully: 'Healers are hosts who patiently and carefully listen to the story of the suffering strangers. Patients are guests who rediscover their selves by telling their story to the one who offers them a place to stay' (p. 89).

Our Own Stories. Our ability to dispense best practices in narrative care is deepened as we learn to take narrative care of ourselves. Narrative care begins at home. It begins with listening to and for and behind our own stories too, listening to what they can tell us about ourselves. It means cultivating a quality of connection with our own inner worlds. It means being present in a compassionate manner to our own questions, our own pain, our own wounds. How can we listen deeply to others in those fleeting spaces that open up between us and serve as agents of development in *their* stories, if we are oblivious to the complexity of our own? How can we avoid foreclosing on them, or 'storyotyping' them (Randall, 1995, p. 57), if we story our own life in constricting ways? How can we facilitate autobiographical learning in *their* lives if we resist such learning ourselves, if we are not asking about the themes and meanings in the narratives by which we understand our life too?

To be agents of autobiographical learning, in whatever situations or for however brief a time, requires an openness to such learning ourselves. This learning can be carried out by many means: by keeping a journal, writing a memoir, making a scrapbook, or simply charting the events that have given our stories their structure and substance to date. In the courses in gerontology that we teach at St Thomas University, we frequently incorporate a narrative component into our assignments: for instance, a lifestory interview with an elderly individual; a reflection paper in which students imagine their own life at 70; guided autobiography groups using selected life-themes; a learning journal in which they take concepts dealt with in class and connect them to their own experience; or an autobiographical essay on their own life story in light of theories that have particularly intrigued them. Such assignments are supremely appropriate in those of our courses that deal directly with the narrative complexity of later life: Narrative Gerontology, Aging and Biography, and Literature and Aging. And, invariably, our students have positive responses: 'I never realized how interesting my own story is, and how much I've learned – and I'm still only 20!' (see Randall, 2002).

Narrative Care in Action. Colleagues in the recreation department of a nearby nursing home, the same one my father announced he would be willing to move into, 'when the time comes,' have embarked on a unique mode of narrative care known as a 'Resident Biography.' It is part of a comprehensive effort to foster a positive narrative environment throughout the institution by a variety of means: reminiscence groups, storytelling circles, conversation corners, scrapbooking parties, not to mention pastoral counselling. As the showpiece of these efforts, the biography program involves extensive interviews with selected residents by specially trained staff, volunteers, family members, or even local high school students. The stories are then presented back to the residents in two main forms: a book filled with their answers to a battery of questions about their life, and a 15-minute video featuring photographs, pieces of their favourite music, and excerpts from their own words – examples of their 'ordinary wisdom,' if you will (Randall & Kenyon, 2001). The video is unveiled at a monthly 'narrative ceremony' held at the nursing home itself, with a resident as honoured guest and a roomful of family, staff, and others in attendance.

The department's director, Daphne Noonan, who holds a master's degree in adult education and is a graduate of our course in narrative gerontology, has written compellingly of how transformative the experience can be for interviewer and interviewee both, and of 'the ripple effect' the program as a whole is having throughout the institution (Noonan, 2011). As the residents' stories are honoured, a quiet culture change is taking place in numerous relationships: resident to staff, resident to family, resident to resident, staff to family, staff to administration, administration to community, and so on. The practice of narrative care is deepening the connections people experience with one another and enriching the environment in which they live or work.

The Medical Arts. Years ago, as a student in Toronto, I would often walk past this imposing structure near the corner of St George and Bloor with the words 'Medical Arts Building' inscribed above the door. The practice of medicine, this phrase reminds us, is both science and art. As a science, medicine has made astonishing strides ahead, developing ever more sophisticated tests and effective medications. Yet, patient by patient, it is an inexact science at best, especially where the elderly are concerned, where normal age-related changes can be so enmeshed with chronic or acute conditions that precise diagnoses and appropriate dosages are challenging to decide. And the end-result of treatment is routinely uncertain: perhaps a temporary prolonging of life, but death itself cannot be stalled forever. This single fact helps to underscore that, ultimately, medicine is an art, arguably the noblest that there is. As many health care professionals knew instinctively before they ever took their training, inspired by the vision of a life devoted to alleviating suffering, attentiveness to bodies and to symptoms is central to the healing arts, but no less so is attentiveness to the stories of the persons in their care.

At the start of his ER drama, my father was seated in a wheelchair, in his pyjamas, while a clerk plied him with questions to get clearer on his symptoms. At one point, a nurse from a nearby cubicle carted in a newborn infant to weigh it on the scales atop the bookcase beside him. I looked at him looking at the baby. He seemed mesmerized. The next day, back at his apartment, I asked him whether part of him (the part not dazed by what was happening to *him*) secretly wished, 'If only I could start all over.' His answer was immediate: *No way*. 'Every person is born into life a blank page,' notes author Christina Baldwin (2005), 'and every person leaves life as a full book' (p. ix). By virtue of his age, Dad's book is all but full. My hope for him, as for other elders like him, is that as he interacts with health care workers in the future, he will sense intuitively that his book is being acknowledged and his story honoured.

REFERENCES

Alheit, P. (1995). Biographical learning: Theoretical outline, challenges, and contradictions of a new approach in adult education. In P. Alheit, A. Bron-Wojciechowska, E. Brugger, & P. Dominice (Eds.), *The biographical approach in European adult education* (pp. 57–74). Vienna: Verband Wiener Voksbildung.

Baldwin, C. (2005). *Story catcher: Making sense of our lives through the power and practice of story.* New York: New World Library.

Bianchi, E. (1991). A spirituality of aging. In L. Cahill & D. Mieth (Eds.), *Aging* (pp. 58–64). London: SCM Press.

Birren, J., & Deutchman, D. (1991). *Guiding autobiography groups for older adults: Exploring the fabric of life.* Baltimore, MD: Johns Hopkins University Press.

Bohlmeijer, E., Kenyon, G., & Randall, W. (2011). Afterword: Towards a narrative turn in health care. In G. Kenyon, E. Bohlmeijer, & W. Randall (Eds.), *Storying later life: Issues, investigations, and interventions in narrative gerontology* (pp. 366–380). New York: Oxford University Press.

Bohlmeijer, E., Valenkamp, M., Westerhof, G., Smit, G., & Cuijpers, P. (2005). Creative reminiscence as an early intervention for depression: Results of a pilot project. *Aging and Mental Health, 9*(4), 302–304.

Brady, M. (1990). Redeemed from time: Learning through autobiography. *Adult Education Quarterly, 41*(1), 43–52.

Butler, R. (2007). Life review. In J.E. Birren (Ed.), *Encyclopedia of gerontology: Age, aging, and the aged.* Vol. 1 (2d ed., pp. 67–72). San Diego, CA: Academic Press. (Original work published 1996.)

Chandler, S., & Ray, R. (2002). New meanings for old tales: A discourse-based study of reminiscence and development in later life. In J. Webster & B. Haight (Eds.), *Critical advances in reminiscence work: From theory to application* (pp. 76–94). New York: Springer.

Charon, R. (2006). *Narrative medicine: Honoring the stories of illness.* New York: Oxford University Press.

Cohen, G. (2005). *The mature mind: The positive power of the aging brain.* New York: Basic Books.

Crisp, J. (1995). Making sense of the stories that people with Alzheimer's tell: A journey with my mother. *Nursing Inquiry, 2,* 133–140.

Cusack, S., & Thompson, W. (2003). *Mental fitness for life: 7 steps to healthy aging.* Toronto: Key Porter Books.

Fireman, G., McVay, T., & Flanagan, O. (Eds.). (2003). *Narrative and consciousness: Literature, psychology, and the brain* (pp. 195–208). New York: Oxford University Press.

Freeman, M. (2010). *Hindsight: The promise and peril of looking backward.* New York: Oxford University Press.

Gold, J. (2002). *The story species: Our life-literature connection.* Markham, ON: Fitzhenry & Whiteside.

Gullette, M. (1997). *Declining to decline.* Chicago: University of Chicago Press.

Hampl, P. (1999). *I could tell you stories: Sojourns in the land of memory.* New York: W.W. Norton.

Holstein, M., & Minkler, M. (2003). Self, society, and the 'new gerontology.' *The Gerontologist, 43*(6), 787–796.

Kennedy, E. (1976). *On becoming a counselor: A basic guide for nonprofessionals.* New York: Crossroads.

Kenyon, G., Bohlmeijer, E., & Randall, W. (Eds.). (2011). *Storying later life: Issues, investigations, and interventions in narrative gerontology.* New York: Oxford University Press.

Kenyon, G., Clark, P., & deVries, B. (Eds.). (2001). *Narrative gerontology: Theory, research, and practice.* New York: Springer.

Kenyon, G., & Randall, W. (1997). *Restorying our lives: Personal growth through autobiographical reflection.* Westport, CT: Praeger.

Labouvie-Vief, G. (2000). Positive development in later life. In T. Cole, R. Kastenbaum, & R. Ray (Eds.), *Handbook of the humanities and aging* (2d ed., pp. 365–380). New York: Springer.

Mader, W. (1995). Thematically guided autobiographical reconstruction: On theory and method of 'guided autobiography' in adult education. In P. Alheit, A. Born-Wojciechowska, E. Brugger, & P. Dominice (Eds.), *The biographical approach in adult education* (pp. 244–257). Vienna: Verband Wiener Volksbildung.

McAdams, D. (1996). Narrating the self in adulthood. In J. Birren, G. Kenyon, J-E. Ruth, J. Schroots, & T. Svensson (Eds.), *Aging and biography: Explorations in adult development* (pp. 131–148). New York: Springer.

McCullough, L. (1993). Arrested aging: The power of the past to make us aged and old. In T. Cole, W. Achenbaum, P. Jakobi, & R. Kastenbaum (Eds.),

Voices and visions of aging: Towards a critical gerontology (pp. 184–204). New York: Springer.

McFadden, S., & Atchley, R. (Eds.). (2001). *Aging and the meaning of time: A multi disciplinary exploration.* New York: Springer.

McLeod, J. (1997). *Narrative and psychotherapy.* London: Sage.

Neisser, U., & Libby, L. (2000). Remembering life experiences. In E. Tulving & F. Craik (Eds.), *The Oxford handbook of memory* (pp. 315–332). New York: Oxford University Press.

Nelson, A. (1994). Researching adult transformation as autobiography. *International Journal of Lifelong Education 13*(5), 389–403.

Noonan, D. (2011). The ripple effect: A story of the transformative nature of narrative care. In G. Kenyon, E. Bohlmeijer, & W. Randall (Eds.), *Storying later life: Issues, investigations, and interventions in narrative gerontology* (pp. 354–365). New York: Oxford University Press.

Nouwen, H. (1976). *Reaching out: The three movements of the spiritual life.* London: Collins.

Randall, W. (1995). *The stories we are: An essay on self-creation.* Toronto: University of Toronto Press.

Randall, W. (2002). Teaching story: The pedagogical potential of narrative gerontology. *Education and Ageing, 17*(1), 55–71.

Randall, W. (2010). The narrative complexity of our past: In praise of memory's sins. *Theory and Psychology, 20*(2), 1–23.

Randall, W., & Kenyon, G. (2001). *Ordinary wisdom: Biographical aging and the journey of life.* Westport, CT: Praeger.

Randall, W., & McKim, E. (2008). *Reading our lives: The poetics of growing old.* New York: Oxford University Press.

Ray, R. (2000). *Beyond nostalgia: Aging and life-story writing.* Charlottesville: University Press of Virginia.

Rowe, J., & Kahn, R. (1998). *Successful aging.* New York: Pantheon.

Rubin, D. (Ed.). (1995). *Remembering our past: Studies in autobiographical memory.* Cambridge: Cambridge University Press.

Ruth, J-E., & Kenyon, G. (1996). Biography in adult development and aging. In J. Birren, G. Kenyon, J-E. Ruth, J. Schroots, & T. Svensson (Eds.), *Aging and biography: Explorations in adult development* (pp. 1–20). New York: Springer.

Schachter-Shalomi, Z., & Miller, R. (1995). *From age-ing to sage-ing: A profound new vision of growing older.* New York: Warner.

Singer, J., & Blagov, P. (2004). The integrative function of narrative processing: Autobiographical memory, self-defining memories, and the life story of identity. In D. Beike, J. Lampinen, & D. Behrend (Eds.), *The self and memory* (pp. 117–138). New York: Psychology Press.

12 Pedagogical BIASes and Clinical Teaching in Medicine

DANIEL D. PRATT, LESLIE SADOWNIK,
AND SANDRA JARVIS SELINGER

Clinicians' teaching roles and responsibilities are diverse and challenging. They teach a variety of learners: undergraduate students, clinical clerks, residents, patients, and families, as well as other health care professionals such as nurses, counsellors, and physiotherapists. They teach in a variety of urgent and non-urgent clinical settings (e.g., emergency departments, outpatient clinics, operating rooms). They may also teach in non-clinical settings: small group seminars or large classroom settings. Across this diversity of pedagogical landscapes, clinicians are expected to teach medical knowledge, procedural skills, clinical reasoning, and professional behaviour and judgment. In chapter 9 in this book, Brookfield speaks similarly to the complexity of clinician's teaching roles.

An abundance of literature describes theoretical foundations and practical guidelines related to teaching and learning in medicine. Some studies have explored teachers' perceptions of their role as educators and provided insights into different approaches to teaching (Mann, Homes, Hayes, Burge, & Weld Viscount, 2001; Morrison, Shapiro, & Harthill, 2005; Stone, Ellers, Homes, Orgren, & Thompson, 2002). Others have elicited students' and residents' opinions regarding effective teacher characteristics (Irby, 1992, 1994). In much of that literature, there is an assumption of generalizability for strategies that influence learning, and, therefore, teaching. For example, clinicians are told that effective teaching and learning is related to involving students in authentic clinical experiences, having students reflect on their learning experience, teaching to students' level of prior knowledge, and ensuring that learning takes place within a supportive environment. For the most part, these strategies are all useful and each might reasonably be assumed to be effective across differences in learners, contexts, and teachers.

However, strategies are only tools. And as with any craft or profession, by separating the tools (strategies) from the craftsperson (teacher) we imply that the tools have the power to facilitate learning. Certainly, some strategies help learning more than others. However, the same teaching strategy can be used by different teachers, or by the same teacher, at different times, but with markedly differing outcomes. A teaching strategy is like a musical instrument awaiting the musical score and the skill of the musician to bring it to life (Pratt, 2005). Therefore, teaching strategies must be interpreted in terms of who wishes to use them, in what settings, with what learners, and for what purposes. This requires critical reflection on the underlying assumptions that guide clinical teaching.

Signature Pedagogies

Just as culture shapes our ways of thinking, valuing, and communicating, it also shapes our perspective on teaching. It is no less true for the 'cultures' or disciplines of medicine. Whether it's family practice or orthopaedics, each specialty has its own 'signature pedagogy' (Shulman, 2005). People are trained (and treated) in ways that convey powerful messages about what is required to become a member of those communities. Through their training, learners adopt the norms of their specialty and take on an identity as a member of that medical community. If they become teachers of others, they may well repeat the patterns of acculturation they experienced – choosing among role models that represent the teacher they want to be. As they do this, they reproduce particular ways of knowing and acting as a particular type of physician. In other words, they go through a process of learning not only what is needed to practice medicine, but also learning how to behave as a clinician and eventually as a teacher.

Pedagogical BIASes

Each medical specialty may also have a dominant set of pedagogical beliefs, intentions, assessments, and strategies, or Pedagogical BIASes:

B – BELIEFS about learners, about the process of learning, about the content or skills to be learned, and beliefs about the role and responsibilities of a teacher;

I – INTENTIONS as to what learners are to learn or what the person teaching them is trying to accomplish;

A – ASSESSMENTS which inform the judgment of learning and learners and the rationale for using those;

S – STRATEGIES or ways in which a clinical teacher combines beliefs,
intentions, and assessments into strategic thinking, and decision-
making, and acting.

Below are five contrasting sets of pedagogical BIASes, each with an
illustrative case of a clinical teacher. Each case represents a perspective
on teaching that illustrates a particular constellation of beliefs, intentions, assessments, and strategies. We want to stress that these cases are
illustrative only and that clinical educators often hold more than one set
of BIASes.

Transmission BIASes in Clinical Teaching

Transmission teachers have a deep commitment to a well-defined body of
knowledge and skill that they believe is essential to practicing medicine.
Effective clinical teaching, from a transmission perspective, helps learners master that body of knowledge and skill. The primary responsibility
of clinical educators is to convey both knowledge and skill to students as
efficiently and effectively as possible. It is the learners' responsibility to
learn that material and develop those skills in their authorized or legitimate forms. There is little ambiguity about what is to be learned, how it
is to be taught, and how it is to be assessed.

Effective Transmission clinical educators take their learners systematically through tasks leading to content mastery: providing clear
objectives, adjusting the pace of delivering content, making efficient
use of time, clarifying misunderstandings, answering questions, providing timely feedback, correcting errors, providing reviews, summarizing
what has been taught, directing them to appropriate resources, setting
high standards for achievement and practice, and developing objective means of assessing learners' knowledge. These teachers are often
deeply dedicated to their specialty and convey that dedication to their
learners.

An Illustrative Case of Transmission BIASes

As a clinical preceptor for gynaecology residents, I offer a four-week
elective in lower genital tract disease. The residents' early specialty
training is primarily hospital based. Consequently, junior residents do

not have a lot of exposure to patients presenting with non-urgent gynaecology problems to an office setting. It is critical that residents learn the basic knowledge and skills required to manage this type of patient. Unfortunately, residents typically arrive on my service with very little background knowledge about these diseases and essentially no practical experience. To facilitate the residents learning of this content area I have taken the following steps:

1. Residents are provided with a set of learning objectives that outline the knowledge and skills that are needed to manage patients. Residents are provided with a standard textbook and a binder of supplemental articles which I expect them to read during the rotation. One afternoon per week is set aside as 'protected time' for the residents to do this reading.
2. I make a point of scheduling a variety of different patients into the clinics so that residents are exposed to a range of disease conditions.
3. I meet with the residents once a week to answer any questions they have about what they are learning and to test them on their knowledge of the material.
4. At the end of the rotation I give the residents a formal written exam. In addition I elicit their formal feedback of the rotation and ask them to identify ways that the rotation could be improved.

Most residents learn a great deal during this rotation and find it a rewarding experience as they can readily see their knowledge and skills improving.

Discussion

Most of us have memorable teachers who were passionate about their discipline or their profession. Like the physician in this case, they could talk with ease and at length about the particulars of their craft or their content. They may have used stories and metaphors that brought the content to life. The clarity of their expectations and delivery may have felt like a gift during a time of academic struggle. Or it may have been the sheer beauty of the material as it was presented. In any case, one of those teachers may have been instrumental to our decision to take up the same discipline. Whether inspiring or boring, all such teachers are convinced of the need to pass along a well-defined, foundational body of knowledge or skill.

This case describes teaching that is based upon a set of predetermined objectives, a well-defined body of knowledge to be learned, concern for precise learning, and efficient and focused teaching of a large volume of material. There is a fundamental belief that a strong knowledge base is the foundation for clinical competence. There is a clear sequencing and ordering of content. Learners are tested to assess the accuracy and sufficiency of their knowledge. This guides the clinician in knowing precisely what is missing and what needs more emphasis, clarification, or direct teaching. Instruction culminates in a formal exam that provides objective assessment and immediate feedback to both the teacher and the learners. There are, of course, other elements in this case that hint at other BIASes, but the dominant view of knowledge, learning, and teaching is typical of a Transmission set of pedagogical BIASes.

Summary of Transmission BIASes

- **Belief:** Learning is facilitated by a clear and organized presentation of information.
- **Intention:** Build a strong base of essential knowledge or skill in learners.
- **Assessment:** Focus on assessing accuracy and sufficiency of learners' knowledge base.
- **Strategy:** High degree of organization, clarity, and structure in the presentation of information.

Apprenticeship BIASes in Clinical Teaching

Effective teaching is also a process of socializing novice clinicians into pre-existing behavioural norms and professional ways of working. The credibility of a teacher in this category of BIASes is based on his/her reputation and skill as a practitioner. Apprenticeship teachers are willing and able to reveal the inner workings of their skilled performance. They are also able to translate that knowledge into a language and set of tasks appropriate to learners' levels of experience. For instance, highly effective teachers here know what their learners can do on their own and where they need guidance and direction. They engage learners within their ZPD, or zone of proximal development (Riber & Carton, 1987). The ZPD is an area of development and maximal learning. It is defined as the difference between what learners can do on their own, without guidance, and what they cannot do, even with guidance. The zone in between those levels of ability is where learning is maximized. As learners mature and become more competent, apprenticeship teachers offer less direction and give more responsibility.

An Illustrative Case of Apprenticeship BIAS

I am a surgeon and I have a variety of learners working with me in the operating room. I am often asked if I think medical students have a legitimate role in the operating room. Yes, I think so. They can help prepare and position the patients; they can learn about establishing a sterile field; and they can be involved in the post-op orders and care of the patient. Initially I engage them in a scrub sink discussion about the medical history of the patient. I briefly describe the procedure that we will be performing and what they can do in the operating room. In the OR, I introduce the student to the operating team and demonstrate how to prep the patient and set up for the operation. Students can be helpful, but you can't assume that they intuitively know what it takes to be a good assistant. This is part of what needs to be demonstrated and explained. The operating room can be an intimidating place for medical students, so it is important to make them feel that they have a functional role in the operation and are not a 'third wheel.'

With residents it's a bit different. Senior residents may have done the procedure before, but again, I can't assume anything. So I begin by asking if they've had an opportunity to do this procedure. Often, there's pressure for the resident to say 'Yes,' even though they may only have assisted. The pressure comes from many sources, but in part it's simply that they want to do it. That's why they are becoming surgeons. If they say they have done the procedure before, I ask them to describe the procedure and the critical points when we want to be most vigilant. This gives me a fair read on where they can work solo and where they will likely need my assistance.

For residents who will be taking the lead in a procedure, I ask them to 'talk out loud' while they are doing the procedure. Some residents are technically good at cutting, but not so good at deciding when to cut and what to watch for as they cut. These judgments are absolutely critical, and I want to hear their reasoning as well as watch their skills.

Once residents are comfortable operating, I direct their attention to the team dynamics within the operating room, and how as a surgeon they are part of a team. Surgery really is a team effort. But it doesn't always look that way. It depends on the surgeon. So this is something they learn by how I behave towards my colleagues in the OR. This can't be learned from a textbook, but it's critical in the operating room. The value of these skills can only be appreciated in the operating room because the decisions they (residents) make have a direct impact on the outcome of the surgery.

Discussion

The Apprenticeship perspective has been dominant in surgical education for over a century. It is founded on the belief that skill, judgment, and confidence are best learned through experience. Many skills are best learned in safe, controlled practise environments where patient safety is not an issue, stress levels are lower, and the difficulty of tasks and skills can be controlled (Guadagnoli & Lee, 2004). But there is no substitute for the mix of people, the pace of coordinated action, and the urgency that characterizes a real operating room. Here the level of task difficulty is not well-defined. It is situational, embedded as it is in the milieu of a dynamic social context and the press of time. Indeed, for much of what is to be learned, context is the teacher (Pratt, Harris, & Collins, 2009). Good Apprenticeship teachers realize this.

In this case, there are several indicators of an Apprenticeship BIAS. This surgeon-educator knows the risks of assuming that what is obvious to him is obvious to learners. This insight points to two important aspects of Apprenticeship: first, the embedded nature of expert knowledge, where experienced clinicians' actions may sometimes render invisible the reasoning and judgment that lies behind those actions; and second, the need to make explicit the many things that are implicit in experienced, professional judgment and actions.

Perhaps most telling in this case is the way the surgeon assesses a resident's zone of proximal development (ZPD), and then monitoring it during the procedure. At the low end there isn't sufficient challenge; at the high end the challenge is too great, and the risk too high – for patient and for learner. The manner in which he assesses this zone, and then activates it during a procedure, are strategic moves that yieldd safer practice and better learning.

All of this is framed within the learning of norms and professional relationships – the culture of surgery and the context of the operating room. An orientation towards the social and cultural aspects of learning and teaching is a central tenet of the Apprenticeship perspective – one which clearly differentiates it from other perspectives. Yet it is often neglected, particularly in contexts that are high risk and pressurized, such as operating rooms, where the entire focus can be on 'doing the case' – for residents this means they are doing the operation; for others it means getting the operative case done. The tension between work and teaching could not be more apparent.

Summary of Apprenticeship BIASes

- **Belief:** Learning is a process of socialization into a community of practice.
- **Intention:** Develop learners' competence and identity as a member of that community.
- **Assessment:** Develop authentic forms of assessment that align with real work.
- **Strategy:** Assess and teach to learner's zone of proximal development (ZPD).

Developmental BIASes in Clinical Teaching

The primary goal of this teaching perspective is to help learners develop increasingly complex and effective forms of reasoning. The key to developing learners' reasoning is a combination of two things: (a) teaching that engages learners with problems or issues and challenging them to move from relatively simple to more complex forms of thinking about those problems or issues; and (b) teachers 'parking' their professional knowledge to allow learners time to construct more complex forms of understanding. To do this, Developmental teachers use problems, cases, and 'why' questions as bridges to transport learners from simpler ways of thinking to new, more complex and sophisticated forms of understanding and reasoning.

Crucial to this way of teaching, is the use of knowledge and expertise in ways that do not undermine the goal of helping learners actively construct their own understanding. From this perspective, *less* (telling) can mean *more* (learning).

An Illustrative Case of Developmental BIAS

I am a family doctor, working in a rural area of our province. For about three months each year, I have either medical students or residents working in my clinical office. For the most part, I really enjoy having them around. They keep me sharp and it's exciting to see the next generation coming along.

With the students, most of what I do is at a pretty basic level. They need to use their basic science learning while also learning to take a history and do a physical exam. But even then it's not straightforward, because it involves making adjustments to different patients. They generally need structure – not a script, but a structure – for thinking about how a chief complaint can lead to a differential diagnosis. So I give them a structure that was given to me. It involves seven things that can help them gather information related to the presenting problem: location, quality, severity, chronology, setting, aggravating or alleviating factors, and manifestations. They can't yet focus their information gathering towards a differential diagnosis, because they don't comprehend the big picture. They've not seen enough patients yet. Everything looks important to them.

With the residents it's different. My goal is similar: that is, to help them learn how to make a good differential diagnosis. But they don't need the formulaic structure that students need; they need to see a wide range of patients and learn to reframe a chief complaint (e.g., pain for last 24 hours) into more general categories of presenting problems (e.g., acute onset of pain). They need to build a repertoire of clinical cases. The vast majority of what I see in the course of a day, is stuff I've seen before. I don't mean that I rush past any patient's chief complaint. But experience does count. So I want to help residents build that kind of clinical experience.

Discussion

A fundamental belief of this perspective is that learning is a search for meaning, based on what one already knows. Prior knowledge is critical to the search for meaning. When learners work alongside experienced physicians, they come with varying degrees of knowledge and capacity to engage in clinical reasoning. Effective Developmental teachers know this and use it to guide their teaching strategies.

The case above is a good illustration of how to be strategic in helping learners at different levels of training develop their clinical reasoning skills. Students come with a foundation of basic science knowledge, but little capacity for clinical reasoning. They need help moving from knowing about diseases to knowing about patients and their presenting conditions. The former does not map readily onto the latter. This physician recognized that and provided a structure for students that would give them the means for gathering and organizing patient-related information With residents he used a different strategy of helping them develop their analytical reasoning (e.g., questioning them about key features) while also helping them build a repertoire of 'pattern recognition.' These two processes are integrated in clinical reasoning (Eva, 2008).

These strategies align with works that describe the developmental stages of clinical reasoning. Initially, learners develop an understanding of the relationship between signs, symptoms, biomedical knowledge, and the pathophysiology of disease. These networks of understanding become more complex and interrelated as learners move on in their training. But in the early stages, they need a conceptual framework to help guide their thinking.

Gradually residents build a repertoire of 'illness scripts' or characteristic features of clinical presentations. These are borne of experience and will form an important part of their clinical reasoning. In the case above, the physician has this stage of learning in mind when he says *they need to see a wide range of patients* ... He is still working on developing clinical reasoning, but now the focus has shifted to pattern recognition, an important part of 'non-analytical' clinical reasoning (Norman, Young, & Brooks, 2007).

Finally, this case illustrates both a strategic approach and multiple, coordinated forms of assessment. With both students and residents, this physician challenges learners to go beyond a decision and into the underlying rationale for their decisions. He holds back his answers until they've given their understanding of the patient's condition. He pushes them to explain what they've ruled out, as well as what they've concluded; what else might be needed to confirm their diagnosis; and why? These questions, along with 'What if ... ' questions, are ways in which he builds a more reliable and valid assessment of the resident (or student) over time and over multiple situations.

Summary of Developmental BIASes

- **Belief:** Learning is a search for meaning and prior knowledge influences that search.
- **Intention:** Develop learners' thinking and reasoning within a specific field or discipline.
- **Assessment:** Use multiple forms and opportunities to assess learners as means of providing low-stakes feedback.
- **Strategy:** Ask learners to reason aloud, ask open-ended questions, and use 'key' features, or 'big' questions to guide learning.

Nurturing BIASes in Clinical Teaching

Those with a nurturing perspective care deeply about their learners and assume that long-term, focused, and persistent effort to achieve comes from the heart as much as it does from the head. They believe that learning is facilitated when: (a) standards for achievement are clear; (b) achievement is acknowledged as a product of the learner's effort and ability rather than the benevolence of a teacher; and (c) the learner's self-esteem and self-concept are not placed at risk. Nurturing teachers provide feedback well in advance of high-stakes accountability and work to develop a trusting relationship in which there can be a balance between academic challenge and emotional support. Nurturing clinical educators do not lower their standards; nor do they excuse learners from doing what is required. Rather, they set challenging but achievable goals within a trusting and supportive learning environment.

An Illustrative Case of Nurturing BIAS[1]

As a pathologist, every day I take care of hundreds of patients whom I never see. I am responsible for interpreting their blood tests correctly and quickly, diagnosing their bone marrow biopsies, and ensuring that their transfusions are safe.

I am also an assistant professor in the Department of Pathology and Laboratory Medicine. Our medical school creates hundreds of new physicians every year, and as a teacher I help each of them care for patients whom I will never meet. Every time these physicians see a patient with abnormal bleeding, every time they encounter a complete blood count or a coagulation result, they will approach these problems with the tools I have given them. Their patients are, in a way, my patients too.

To care for their patients, medical students need to learn thousands of complex facts during their four years of training. They will not get very many of these facts from me. What they will get, whether they are in a lecture hall of 250 students or sitting next to me one-on-one at the microscope, is a way to think about mechanisms of disease. I teach my students how to approach patients with hematologic illness by imagining what is going on at the molecular and cellular and tissue level. In short, I teach my students not what to think but how to think. I help my students build a mental foundation, on which they can place each of the details they so painstakingly memorize. My hope is that, at three in the morning on some future night when on call, that foundation will be there to support them.

I make it a point to get to 'connect' with each of my students. To connect with my students, I work very hard to understand what they already know – how much, or how little. It is all very well to have learning objectives and exit competencies, to know where the students have to finish their educational journey, but even the clearest map is useless if where you are right now is a mystery. Knowing where to start, which amounts to having 'educational empathy,' is sometimes challenging: clearly, any medical school class with artists and writers sitting next to nurses and PhD scientists is bound to have wide variations in background knowledge. I make a real effort to find where the students are, to know what they know, and to guide each of them to their destination – challenging and supporting them along the way.

Discussion

On first read, this case seems as though it might be an instance of a Developmental teacher. This teacher believes in the importance of the prior knowledge that his students and residents bring to their learning. He works hard to understand what they already know – how much, or how little. This is part of 'connecting' with his students. He calls it having 'educational empathy.' This is a strategic move; that is, to know where to begin before deciding how to take students further into the realm of reasoning about disease mechanisms.

His intention is also similar to what we've seen in the Developmental perspective. He is concerned with developing a form of clinical reasoning, a way to think about mechanisms of disease. He will not be teaching them the myriad of facts they will acquire through their training. He teaches his students not what to think, but how to think.

Nurturing and Developmental teaching perspectives are not mutually exclusive; there is some overlap. However, there is a difference, and it is most evident in a deeper read of this philosophy of teaching. Throughout the statement there is a deep concern for students and patients. He talks about 'connecting' with his students not just as a means of facilitating learning, but as a way of connecting with and relating to them. It's the learners that are the subject, not their past knowledge; and it's the learners he wants to connect with. Through these connections, he is reaching out to patients he will never see, but he nonetheless considers them 'his patients.' This reveals a different kind of pedagogical BIAS – one that brings the person/student/patient into focus as he talks about his orientation to teaching.

There is a pervasive sense of concern and caring that characterizes this pathologist's approach to teaching. He does not focus on content; nor is it sufficient to teach reasoning. He wants his teaching to reach forward, through the students and into the lives of patients – his patients. His opening line speaks volumes: As a pathologist, every day I take care of hundreds of patients whom I never see. 'I take care of ...' This is not a passive statement about teaching; it's an active statement of caring. This is a different kind of perspective and set of BIASes. It is no less effective, nor is it more effective. It's just different. But in the person of this man, it is a very effective approach to teaching.

Summary of Nurturing BIASes

- **Belief:** Learning is both emotional and intellectual.
- **Intention:** Develop self-efficacy and agency in learners.
- **Assessment:** Build positive and trusting relationships with learners to facilitate constructive feedback and assessment.
- **Strategy:** Balance high expectations and challenge with provision of support.

Social Reform BIASes in Clinical Teaching

Effective Social Reform teaching seeks to change society or the profession in substantive ways. From this point of view, the object of teaching is the collective as well as the individual. Highly effective clinical educators with this as their teaching perspective awaken students to values and ideologies that are embedded in texts and common practices within health care more broadly. Social Reform educators challenge the status quo and encourage learners to consider how individuals (e.g., patients, physicians, nurses) are positioned and constructed in particular discourses and practices. This comes close to the challenging perspective offered by Egan early on in this book.

To do so, they deconstruct common practices to reveal ways in which those practices appear 'normal' but actually perpetuate conditions that are unacceptable. Their teaching focuses not only on specific knowledge or practices, but also on how knowledge and ways of practising have been created, by whom, and for what purposes. Texts are interrogated for both what is said and what is not said; what is included and what is excluded; who is represented and who is omitted from the dominant discourse. Medical students are encouraged to take a critical stance to give them power to take social action to improve their own lives and the lives of others. Though central to Social Reform, critical deconstruction is not an end in itself; if deconstruction does not serve to improve society or the profession, it is not considered effective teaching or learning.

An Illustrative Case of Social Reform BIAS

I teach surgical residents in a trauma centre. Recently, we had a case involving a woman whose car was hit by a drunk driver. She was brought by paramedics to the emergency department, unconscious and in serious condition. The other driver was brought to the same emergency with a number of injuries. He was conscious but disoriented.

The woman survived the night, but was comatose and had a poor prognosis. The man was treated for a number of non-fatal orthopedic injuries, but kept overnight in hospital for observation and monitoring. The next day, at the morning case conference, I presented this case and asked the residents how they would discuss each patient's condition with their respective worried families.

After some discussion, I added information given to me by the officers that attended the scene: the man had been drinking and had a number of driving-while-impaired charges. On this occasion, he was impaired and had been driving without a license. I asked the residents if this would affect their discussion with each patient's family. Most felt it would not.

I then asked the residents where their responsibility as health care providers ends. Does it end with the death of the woman? Does it end with the discharge of patients? I challenged them to consider the relationship between alcohol and drugs and the trauma cases we see, including this one that was the result of impaired driving. We discussed the magnitude of the problem in Canada – the number of deaths, injuries, and cost to society. Some of them were really engaged in the discussion; others were not at all convinced that their responsibility extended beyond the care of the injuries incurred.

I strongly believe that physicians need to see how individual health and mortality is part of more complex societal issues – in this case the relationship between alcohol and driving. As physicians, we often see the tragic end result of society's illnesses, and I have a responsibility to advocate for changes that will improve the bigger picture of health.

Discussion

Social Reform is the most difficult set of pedagogical BIASes to describe because it has no single, defining set of assessments or strategies. Indeed, highly effective Social Reform teachers have much in common with other effective educators. They are clear and organized in their teaching; they bring learners into diverse communities of practice; they ask probing questions and use powerful metaphors that help learners bridge prior knowledge and new concepts; and they work hard to respect and promote the dignity and self-efficacy of their learners.

Social Reform teachers, however, hold a belief that differentiates them from other perspectives. With strong conviction, they believe that teachers are obligated to address broader social issues that perpetuate injustice, inequity, or simply something that is wrong in society. As teachers, therefore, they work towards social change, not simply individual learning. It is the collective as much as the individual that is the object of their teaching. Social Reform teachers are unequivocal and clear about what changes are desired and necessary. They see themselves as instruments of social change, and are known amongst their colleagues and students as advocates for the changes they wish to bring about in society.

In the case above, there was no question where to begin: each patient was assessed and managed with all due diligence and care. That was the first priority. However, as the teacher pointed out in the case conference the next morning, that was not the end of the responsibility for a trauma surgeon. The questions posed to the residents about their responsibility clearly raise issues that are not part of the usual discussion in morning conferences. And many, if not most, other trauma surgeons would likely question whether it is even appropriate to pose such questions to residents. It is common for Social Reform teachers to have colleagues question their focus on issues considered beyond the bounds of normal practices in medicine. But that is exactly what this teacher is committed to doing: that is, challenging what is 'normal' and taken-for-granted in the practice of medicine. This Social Reform teacher is not alone in this, but is most likely in the minority.

Summary of Social Reform BIASes

- **Belief:** Learning and knowledge are saturated with values related to power, privilege, and authority.

- **Intention:** Develop competent learners, but point out ways in which normal practices can unwittingly perpetuate something that is 'wrong.'
- **Assessment:** Look for indication of learners' commitment to changing professional practices in ways that address societal problems.
- **Strategy:** Provoke a state of discomfort with the status quo in learners.

Conclusions and Implications

In fulfilling their professional duties, clinical teachers carry the dual obligation of educating the next generation while also providing safe and compassionate care to patients. This duality of role and obligation is not made easier by debates about what constitutes the best or most effective model of clinical teaching. Any search for the Holy Grail of teaching will contribute more confusion than clarity when it comes time to teach.

Pedagogical BIASes are a part of our being and thus the lenses through which we view our students and our educational work. They are the places from which we frame each situation and then make choices and judgments about what to do, what worked or didn't work, and what to do next time. As such, they are relatively stable characteristics of our being. In the deepest sense, they represent epistemological positions with different underlying assumptions about knowledge, learning, and the appropriate roles of learners and teachers.

Yet, it is not sufficient to simply identify our pedagogical BIASes. The power and purpose of each set of BIASes lies not in its eloquence or its fit with some current fad about teaching, but in its ability to reveal what is hidden but essential to understanding someone's teaching. At their best, they are a map to the deeper structures of a clinical educator's assumptions and commitments, revealing the logic and justification behind the acts of teaching. However, across all pedagogical BIASes there is one foundational belief that characterizes effective teachers: they truly believe that what is learned is more important than what is taught. It could not be otherwise for them to be effective.

NOTE

1 We acknowledge, with thanks, Dr. Jason Ford for this case.

REFERENCES

Eva, K. (2008). The cross-cutting edge: Striving symbiosis between medical education research and related disciplines. *Medical Education, 42*(10), 950–951.

Guadagnoli, M.A., & Lee, T.D. (2004). Challenge point: A framework for conceptualizing the effects of various practice conditions in motor learning. *Journal of Motor Behaviour, 36*(2), 212–224.

Irby, D.M. (1992). How attending physicians make instructional decisions when conducting teaching rounds. *Academic Medicine, 67*(10), 630–638.

Irby, D.M. (1994). What clinical teachers in medicine need to know. *Academic Medicine, 69*(5), 333–342.

Mann, K.V., Homes, D.B., Hayes, V.M., Burge, F.I., & Weld Viscount, P. (2001). Community family medicine teachers' perceptions of their teaching role. *Medical Education, 35*(3), 278–285.

Morrison, E.H., Shapiro, J.F., & Harthill, M. (2005). Resident doctors' understanding of their roles as clinical teachers. *Medical Education, 39*(2), 137–144.

Norman, G., Young, Y., & Brooks, L. (2007). Non-analytical models of clinical reasoning: The role of experience. *Medical Education, 41*(12), 1140–1145.

Pratt, D.D. (2005). Teaching. In L.M. English (Ed.), *International encyclopedia of adult education.* New York: Palgrave Macmillan.

Pratt, D.D., Harris, P., & Collins, J.B. (2009). The power of one: Looking beyond the teacher in clinical instruction. *Medical Teacher, 31*(2), 133–137.

Rieber, R.W., & Carton, A.S. (Eds.). (1987). *The collected works of L.S. Vygotsky.* New York: Plenum Press.

Shulman, L. (2005). Signature pedagogies in the professions. *Daedalus, 134*(3), 52–59.

Stone, S., Ellers, B., Homes, D., Orgren, R., Qualters, D., & Thompson, J. (2002). Identifying oneself as a teacher: The perceptions of preceptors. *Medical Education, 36*(2), 180–185.

13 Reflective Practice for Allied Health: Theory and Applications

ELIZABETH ANNE KINSELLA, MARIE-ÈVE
CATY, STELLA NG, AND KAREN JENKINS

This chapter offers an introduction to reflective practice in allied health from both theoretical and practical perspectives. Reflective practice is recognized as an important dimension of adult learning, and as an approach to lifelong learning and professional development in the professions. The chapter is aimed at future and current practitioners and written by an occupational therapist, a speech language pathologist, an audiologist, and a registered nurse. It begins with a discussion of reflective practice and an examination of different types of reflection, followed by three case studies. The case studies illuminate how reflective practice may be used to advance adult learning and professional development in the health professions. Finally, ways of becoming a reflective practitioner are highlighted, as well as some of the potential benefits, challenges, and enablers to reflective practice.

An Introduction to Reflective Practice

Amidst the speed in which we live and work, there has been a lack of acknowledgement of the importance of reflection and its significance for the cultivation of professional knowledge that begins in practice. In response to this issue, reflective practice was popularized by Donald Schön (1983) in his seminal and thought provoking book, *The Reflective Practitioner: How Professionals Think in Action.* In this book, Schön explores sources of professional knowledge and inquires into the kinds of knowledge important for successful professional practice. He posits that there is a kind of knowledge that is distinct from the propositional knowledge presented in textbooks and scientific papers, a knowledge embedded in professional practice itself. In Schön's (1983) words, 'this knowing-in-practice is largely tacit; thus competent practitioners usually know more than they can say' (p.viii). Schön's work (1983, 1987) calls for an inquiry into the epistemology of practice, and attends to, documents, and researches case studies that illuminate knowing-in-practice. Schön describes reflective practice as the capacity of practitioners to engage in reflection on the knowing embedded in their performance, which involves reflection on their own actions in practice. According to Schön, such reflection can occur in the midst of action or after the action. In his classic case studies, Schön (1983) revealed how artful practitioners use reflection to learn from experience and to improve their professional practices. He also revealed how practitioners use reflection to cope with the unique, uncertain, and conflicted situations of practice. Schön (1983, 1987, 1992, 1994) published a number of deeply influential books about the processes of becoming and educating reflective practitioners. He came to define reflective practice as 'a dialogue of thinking and doing through which I become more skillful' (1987, p. 31). Reflective practice may be seen as a way for professionals to learn through reflection on their experience, as a way to generate knowledge in and from practice, as a means to acknowledge practitioner experiential knowledge as significant, and as an approach to negotiating the challenging complexities of professional practice.

Reflective practice is attentive to the intelligence revealed through professional performance, what Schön calls 'knowing-in-action' (Kinsella, 2007b). It calls for increased consideration of the knowledge emanating from and generated through practice. One way to think about knowing-in-action is to consider a senior practitioner charged with educating a junior practitioner in a clinical context. The senior practitioner possesses significant knowledge, which is conveyed through the instructions, knowledge, insights, and rationale for action offered to the junior practitioner; but it is also conveyed through intelligent action, through the senior practitioners' knowing-in-action, what he or she actually does, and this knowledge may be more tacit. One could consider this knowledge to be a mixture of different types of knowledge, including 'knowing that' – or propositional knowledge, as well as 'knowing-how' – a kind of knowledge that is not usually found in books but rather is revealed in intelligent action (Kinsella, 2007b; Polanyi, 1967; Ryle, 1949; Schön, 1983).

Schön's writing on reflective practice emerged just prior to the widespread adoption of the evidence-based practice movement (Sackett, Straus, Richardson, Rosenberg, & Haynes, 2000) and the calls for increased accountability of autonomous professionals (Greiner &

Knebel, 2003; Higgs, Richardson, & Dahlgren, 2004) in allied health care. Yet Schön was concerned with what he perceived as an excessive emphasis on technical rationality in conceptions of professional knowledge (Kinsella, 2007a). Schön (1987) defined technical rationality as holding that 'professionals are instrumental problem solvers who select technical means best suited to particular purposes' (p. 3). In this conception 'rigorous professional practitioners solve well formed instrumental problems by applying theory and technique derived from systematic preferably scientific knowledge' (p. 3). Schön problematized the predominance of technical knowledge over practice-based knowledge and highlighted an emerging crisis of confidence in professional knowledge. He suggested that the crisis of professional knowledge could be overcome in part by 'flipping' technical rationality 'on its head' (Kinsella, 2007a, p. 105). In other words, Schön believed that rather than focusing solely on technical rationality and research-based knowledge, professions could benefit from a redirection of attention to practice-based knowledge. Some scholars of reflection purport that Schön sets up a dichotomy between practice-based versus research-based knowledge (Fenstermacher, 1988; Moon, 1999), while others contend that Schön does not dismiss science or technique as irrelevant but rather that he draws attention to dimensions that have been under-represented in light of technical rationality (Grimmett & Erickson, 1988; Kinsella, 2007a). In other words, scientific and practice-based knowledge may fruitfully be viewed as complementary rather than dichotomous (Kinsella, 2007a; Mantzoukas, 2007; Mantzoukas & Watkinson, 2008).

Types of Reflection

In The Reflective Practitioner, Schön (1983) highlighted how reflection-in-action is a frequently overlooked means of developing knowledge important for professional practice. Further, Schön (1983, 1987) highlighted the significance of reflection-on-action for practitioner knowledge. Two additional types of reflection are also proposed as important for reflective practitioners: anticipatory reflection (Kinsella, 2000; van Manen, 1991) and critical reflection (Brookfield, 1998, 2000).

Reflection-in-Action

Reflection-in-action takes place within professional practice in the midst of professional activity. It is often stimulated when practitioners apply their theoretical/professional knowledge and are met with an unexpected outcome (Kinsella, 2000). Schön (1983) describes reflection-in-action as the ability to 'think on your feet' (p. 54).

The stages of reflection-in-action have been described by Donald Schön (1987) and summarized by Kinsella (2000). Reflection-in-action usually begins with a dilemma or a surprise; an event or occurrence in practice that does not go as expected. This unexpected situation causes the practitioner to reflect in the midst of the action itself. An example from nursing practice involves a nurse who was giving an elderly client an intramuscular injection. In the course of administering the injection she realized that the muscle was severely atrophied. She reflected that she was unable to administer the injection fully into the muscle in the manner in which she had been taught, and that if she did so the needle would hit the patient's bone. The nurse reflected on the event in the moment and recognized that she needed to rethink her approach to administering the injection in such a way that the medicine would be released into the muscle and wouldn't touch the bone. She reflected on her knowing-in-action, how she usually gives intramuscular injections successfully, and rethinks her usual course of action. The nurse had already begun the injection and in the midst of the action she engaged in on the spot experimentation and adjusted the depth of the insertion of the needle, taking into account the size of the muscle mass, in order to avoid reaching the bone, and in order to release the medication into the muscle.

In the above example the nurse adjusts her action in the midst of performing the skill of giving an injection. Schön (1987) describes reflection in the midst of action as 'action-present – a period of time, variable with the context, during which we can still make a difference to the situation at hand; our thinking serves to reshape what we are doing while we are doing it' (p. 26). A practitioner who is overly confident, and fails to recognize dilemmas in practice or to engage in reflection-in-action 'may miss important opportunities to think about what he is doing' (Schön, 1983 p. 61).

Reflection-on-Action

Reflection-on-action occurs after the event and is a kind of retrospective thinking or looking back on the situation/event to examine it anew. Reflection-on-action allows the practitioner to make sense of actions taken, to consider the context and consequences of those actions, and to intentionally learn from the experience. Thus, reflection-on-action can lead to a change in future action.

Reflection-on-action can occur through a variety of approaches. For example, a student clinician could review a video of her interactions with a client. A professional or student practitioner could keep a journal in which she records reflective thoughts at the end of each day of a clinical position or practicum (Moon, 1999, 2004). A mentor and mentee could have a reflective conversation after a clinical appointment (Johns, 2002).

Reflection-on-action is a way to explicitly engage in professional development, drawing from practical experience as the main source of knowledge (Kinsella, 2000). Reflection-on-action is involved in the process of experiential learning, where it serves to help us learn or create knowledge from experience (Kolb, 1984). Reflection-on-practice allows us to look back at our practices, to critique them, and to modify our future practices based on the new knowledge that has been created based on reflection upon the prior experience.

Anticipatory Reflection

Anticipatory reflection is a type of reflection that occurs prior to action in professional practice. 'Anticipatory reflection enables practitioners to deliberate about possible alternatives, decide on courses of action, plan the kinds of things we need to do, and anticipate the experiences we and others may have as a result of expected events or of our planned actions' (van Manen, 1991, p. 101). Most often professionals engage in anticipatory reflection without thinking about it (Kinsella, 2001).

Anticipatory reflection provides an opportunity for allied health professionals to pause and reflect on previous experiences similar to the experience at hand. It affords an opportunity to reflect on what went well and what did not go well, and to prepare for the upcoming task or interaction, in order to improve health care practice and patient outcomes (Kinsella, 2001).

Critical Reflection

Critical reflection in practice involves encouraging allied health practitioners to examine assumptions, including beliefs, values, social, and systemic structures (Brookfield, 1998; Mezirow, 1990; White, Fook, & Gardiner, 2006). Critical reflection involves an examination of how such dimensions influence our daily professional practices. According to Brookfield (2000), critically reflective practitioners examine power relations, and consider how ideological perspectives shape the practice contexts in which they work. Allied health practitioners who engage in critical reflection may uncover power dynamics and recognize hegemonic assumptions: that is, assumptions which shape practice in ways that may not be in practitioners' or clients' best interests. In chapter 9 in this book Brookfield delves further into how to shape teaching practice that is in the students' interests.

Critical reflection allows allied health practitioners to stand outside of their practice and to see their decisions and actions from a broader perspective (Brookfield, 1998). Thus, a critically reflective practitioner may be more likely to identify externally imposed limitations to their practices, and subsequently impart change.

Conceptions of critical reflection are compatible with Schön's work, although Schön did not describe critical reflection. Indeed, many allied health practitioners who engage in reflective practice report coming to more critically reflective insights over time. Placing a critical lens on reflection inherently shifts the focus and purpose of reflection and has important implications for understanding and advancing professional practice.

Reflective Practice Case Studies

The following cases are intended to (a) illuminate the distinct types of reflection previously described, and (b) highlight the complex processes of reflective practice. Illuminating occasions for reflection so distinctly, however, barely signals that most reflective moments in professional practice are ephemeral episodes disappearing as quickly as they arise in a flow of simultaneous actions (Schön, 1992). Moments of reflection are rarely as distinct from one another as they are presented in the following cases. Readers are invited to review these short case studies before considering further issues and challenges of becoming a reflective practitioner highlighted in the concluding section of the chapter.

Occupational Therapy: Reflective Practice Case Study

Critical Incident: Mark is an occupational therapy student, who is working with an occupational therapist in community mental health as part of an Assertive Community Treatment (ACT) Team. He and his supervising therapist have just arrived at a client's home and no one is answering the door. The client has a history of drug and alcohol abuse and rarely leaves his home. The therapist is concerned that perhaps he has passed out or overdosed on substances, and worried that he may need medical attention. The supervising therapist instructs the student to crawl through the window and open the door so that they can check on the client and ensure his safety.

Reflection-in-Action

Mark begins to move towards the window. As he is moving he recognizes a nagging feeling in his stomach, and he begins to think about the implications of crawling through the window. He wonders: Is this legal? Could I be charged with break and enter? What if there is a man inside, and he is concerned about seeing a stranger in his home? Would he be angry? Could I be hurt? Mark also reflects on his relationship with his supervisor; he respects and trusts her opinion and he is confident she would not steer him wrong. He wonders if he is at risk of ruining the relationship with her if he refuses.

In response to these reflections Mark stops at the window and rethinks his course of action. Mark informs the therapist that he is not really comfortable entering the home because (a) he doesn't know the client and it may frighten the client to see a stranger in his home, (b) he doesn't know the hospital policies or if he is covered to do this, and (c) he is worried about the legal implications – could this been seen as break and enter? His supervising therapist apologizes; she indicates that she has a long history with this client, and that they have a trusting relationship. The ACT Team has a signed permission from the client on file to enter his home if he is not responding to the door. She has a key to the house but has forgotten it on this day. However, the therapist agrees that upon reflection the best course of action is for her to enter the home rather than him, and that perhaps the best way to do so is to return to the office and get the key that is on file.

Reflection-on-Action

As it turns out, the client is found unconscious and the therapist calls 911. He appears to have overdosed on an unknown substance. Medical treatment in this instance saves the man's life. Both the therapist and the student reflect on the event. The student reflects that he has learned about a whole side of practice he could never have imagined, and that he is glad that he had the courage to speak up to his therapist and that they were able to intervene to save the client's life. The therapist reflects on the student's comments and recognizes that his concerns were very legitimate. She is glad that she was the one to enter the house, and that the client received the medical treatment he required. She realizes that she placed the student in an awkward position and that in the future she would be more conscious about the implications of such a request with a student.

Anticipatory Reflection

The therapist reflects on how she will change her expectations with future students. She also reflects on how the ACT team had good foresight in developing a contract with the client concerning entering the house. The therapist reflects that they were fortunate to get to the client on time in this instance, and decides, at least in the short term, to bring the key when she sees this client in case of a future event of this nature.

Critical Reflection

Both the student and the therapist reflect critically on the power relationship in the student/ clinician relationship. The therapist in this instance did not insist that Mark enter the home, and did not penalize him on his fieldwork evaluation, which could have been an outcome had she not been open to rethinking her own assumptions and cognizant of the therapist/student power relations.

Speech Language Pathology: Reflective Practice Case Study

Mr C, 76 years old, had survived a laryngectomy (removal of the voice box) against all odds. Mr C experienced several post-surgery medical complications which resulted in an extended stay at the hospital. Voiceless as a result of the surgery, he was trained by the speech-language pathologist (SLP) to use an intraoral artificial larynx in order to provide him with a means to communicate verbally. This device restores speech through the use of an external, electronic voicing source that is directed into the oral cavity and articulated into speech production.

The speech device was modified to overcome some challenges pertaining to hand dexterity. Despite Mr C's limitations, training efforts were made to foster his positive attitude towards the use of the intraoral artificial larynx. This was especially important since the SLP knew well how laryngectomized patients may become withdrawn or feel isolated by their inability to speak. Mr C committed to speech therapy sessions, though he became quickly fatigued and was sometimes discouraged. His wife, who was at his bedside daily, often attended therapy sessions but sometimes opted for a rest instead.

Critical Incident: When invited to attend an interprofessional meeting regarding Mr C, the SLP was surprised to hear that Mr C had been deemed to be non-compliant with his rehabilitative treatment and that his wife had refused to be involved in providing care. It was the first time that all the professionals involved were invited to such a 'team' meeting. Mr C and his wife were expected to attend the meeting as well as community care team members. Everyone's contribution was requested in order to resolve the issues which were deemed to be preventing Mr C from being discharged from the hospital.

Anticipatory Reflection

The SLP reviewed her professional record, which suggested that Mr C was making progress using his speech device. From the SLP's perspective nothing was preventing Mr C from being discharged from the hospital since she could arrange outpatient service for him to complete his training. In therapy, his wife was supporting him in his effort to learn to speak using an electronic artificial larynx. She could assist him to use it at home. The SLP did not 'see' the couple in the same way as the rest of the team; that is, as non-compliant.

Framing the Problem

During the team meeting, when Mr C's wife burst into tears upon hearing that she was preventing the discharge of her husband, the team realized she was exhausted. It became clear that the couple needed additional support to transit back to their home. The whole team reframed the issue of non-compliance to an issue of a need for respite for the caregiver. A respite care facility was sought for Mr C so that his wife could rest. Community care team members would become involved later, when Mr C would return home.

Reflection-in-Action

The SLPs course of action now changed; she was now concerned about sustaining Mr C's speech rehabilitation at the respite care facility and later his communication with the community care team who would visit him at home. The community care team members attending the meeting were eager to understand how to best communicate with Mr C. The SLP suggested communication strategies and prepared written instructions for them and for the caregivers at the respite care facility.

Reflection-on-Action

The SLP reflected upon the challenge of communication and conflict resolution between a professional team and a patient and his family. She wondered whose responsibility it was to ensure that the lines of communication were clear, and to support the family members of patients.

Critical Reflection

The SLP reflected on how the absence of speech can lead people to think that a patient has reduced competence or is less capable of understanding. Without words, actions can be easily misinterpreted. She wondered if the team was sensitive to the vulnerability of Mr C and the resulting power imbalance between the team and the couple. She also considered how to empower laryngectomized patients to become active participants in their health care.

Audiology: Reflective Practice Case Study

Critical Incident: Sue is a new audiologist nearing the end of her first year of practice. An infant has been referred to her through the province's Infant Hearing Program. The infant had previously been screened for hearing loss, at which time she passed the tests. However, the infant has returned for further testing due to a number of high-risk factors that were unknown at the time of the initial hearing screening, but later identified at a medical appointment. These factors suggested that the infant would have a higher likelihood for hearing loss.

Sue conducts an assessment and identifies a severe-to-profound sensorineural hearing loss. Upon informing the parents of her assessment findings, Sue realizes that the parents are holding on to the normal hearing results obtained months earlier. Typically at this point, Sue would explain results and options to the parents, but she quickly realizes that they are not ready to hear this information, and sets up a follow-up appointment that will involve a support worker and other relevant professionals.

Reflection-in-Action

The audiologist realized that the parents of the infant were not ready to have a conversation about hearing loss, and chose to postpone any discussions to a later date. The audiologist's espoused theory was that early intervention is of utmost importance, and that delaying intervention – whether it be the process of acquiring amplification or beginning the steps towards a sign-language approach – can have a significant impact on the social and educational future of the infant. However, Sue recognized that the parents seemed to be in denial, and that it would be overwhelming and potentially detrimental to push the matter on this day, and she acted accordingly.

Reflection-on-Action

After the family leaves, Sue feels conflicted, and contacts her mentor, an experienced pediatric audiologist. Together, they go over the assessment results, re-affirm that Sue has done the best assessment that she could, discuss the family's reactions, and reflect on the difficult road ahead. They reflect on the results that were previously communicated to the parents regarding their infant's normal hearing at birth, and consider areas for improvement in the infant hearing screening process to assist in obtaining an accurate case history to identify at-risk infants. They reflect on ways to communicate realistic expectations, and educate parents with high-risk infants without unnecessarily scaring them.

Critical Reflection

As the case progresses, Sue becomes frustrated by the parents' continued resistance to accept the findings of the assessment and the delayed decision-making on behalf of the child. Sue speaks with the support worker and reflects on the challenging decisions that the family faces; she realizes that her own assumptions about what the infant needs may not align with the family's values and beliefs. Further, societal stigmatization and debates between advocates for the oral/aural language approaches and Deaf Culture and sign-language approaches make it even more challenging for parents to make a life-shaping decision for their very young child. Sue realizes that although, up to this point in her career, decisions of this nature have been seemingly more straightforward, family values and their interactions with societal influences can add a layer of complexity to a situation.

Becoming a Reflective Practitioner

The cases above offer examples of reflective practice in the context of allied health professions while illuminating different types of reflection. The cases show how reflective practice may contribute to adult learning and professional development in the health professions, with the assumption that ongoing reflection and learning in professional life contributes to improved outcomes for clients in the health care context.

The next section considers some key dimensions of becoming a reflective practitioner revealed in the previous case studies. These include: attention to the indeterminate zones of practice, the potential of critical incidents to invite reflection, the importance of framing the problem through reflection, the use of reflective writing, and the use theories of practice as a means of professional development and lifelong learning.

Indeterminate Zones of Practice. Reflection often begins in what Schön (1983, 1987) referred to as the indeterminate zones of practice: those dimensions of practice that are confusing, messy, uncertain, or laden with conflicts of values, goals, purposes, or interests. Reflection is seen to begin when practitioners are confronted with such indeterminate zones of practice: those dimensions that are not clear-cut, and when there is an outcome or event that doesn't meet the practitioner's expectations. In the previous case studies, this could be seen in Mark's reflections about what his preceptor was asking him to do. Such events can be disorienting or confusing, yet these may be the moments when a practitioner considers anew a clinical situation or brings a fresh mind to the situation at hand.

Critical Incidents. Critical incidents in professional life are another means by which reflection is frequently fostered. Benner (2001), a scholar of nursing education, describes critical incidents as an approach for eliciting reflective thought. A critical incident is a thought-provoking clinical experience in which one's practice made an exceptional difference to a patient, went unusually well or unexpectedly, was especially extraordinary or demanding, or captured the 'quintessence' of one's professional mandate (p. 300). Reflection upon a critical incident might encompass reflection upon the incident's context, the practitioners' concerns at the time, the thoughts and feelings experienced during and following the incident or experience. The cases above began with a critical incident from an allied health practitioner's life, and reveal how

such incidents require practitioner reflection if they are to be successfully navigated.

Framing the Problem. Framing the problem through reflection encompasses how the practitioner selectively attends to certain variables within
a clinical situation in order to determine the problems to which he/she
will attend. The agency of the practitioner, the capacity to choose how to
think and act, allows him or her to critically select the problematic characteristic of a situation and to frame the issues and set the boundaries of
the situation. As noted by Schön (1987), problems do not present themselves to the practitioners as givens; rather, they must be constructed
from the materials of problematic situations which are puzzling, trou-
bling, and uncertain. Schön (1983) writes that 'professional practice
has at least as much to do with finding the problem as with solving the
problem found' (p. 18). The setting of the problem, or the framing of
the problematic situation is as important, if not more important, for the
reflective practitioner, as the actions he/she takes towards resolution
of the problem (Schön, 1994). For example, one previous case study
attempted to make explicit how practitioners within a team framed a
particular problem, and how such framing was crucially implicated in
the process of resolution.

Reflective Writing. One means by which practitioners frequently engage
in reflective practice and learn about their own professional practices
is through reflective writing. Writing acts as a tool to assist practitioners
to reflect on their thinking and actions in practice. The very process of
writing compels practitioners to become more aware of what they are
thinking, feeling, and experiencing (Boud, 2001). Reflective writing in
professional practice often takes the form of reflective journals; however,
it may also include learning logs, diaries, autobiographies, reflective stories, and poetry (Bolton, 2010). Bolton describes writing as a reflective
process whereby practitioners take responsibility for their own actions by
exploring complex professional practice issues such as professional values and ethics. Writing can encourage practitioners to reflect at a deeper
level, allowing them to make sense of and better understand complex
situations.

In the audiology reflective practice case study, Sue struggled with her
own feelings regarding the parents' resistance to accept the test findings. Sue may have benefited from a written exploration of her feelings and judgments regarding this family. Reflective writing may have

offered Sue a way of seeing her practice differently, and enabled her to further explore her own judgments. Actively reflecting-in-action and/or reflecting-on-action (Schön 1983, 1987) through writing enables practitioners to become researchers of their own practice, providing them with data in the form of written text with which to question, interrogate, and explore unclear or messy situations in practice and to engage in a deeper, transformative learning process (Jenkins, 2011).

Theories of Practice. Another dimension of reflective practice that is frequently overlooked is the significance of practitioners' theories of practice, in terms of the actions they undertake in practice. According to Argyris and Schön (1992), practitioners hold theories of practice that consist of (a) espoused theories, and (b) theories-in-use. Espoused theories are the principles and beliefs that practitioners can easily talk about when asked to describe their everyday work life. Another way to understand espoused theories is to ask a practitioner how he/she would behave under certain circumstances (Argyris & Schön). Espoused theories are the principles of action that practitioners give allegiance to and communicate with, and they often carry the profession's explicit principles and values. Theories-in-use, on the other hand, are contained within the practitioner's actions and are demonstrated in what he/she actually does (Kinsella, 2001). They are the principles or theories that actually govern professional actions. The practitioner may not be able to articulate his or her theory-in-use and may not even be conscious of it. As underlying beliefs are revealed through action, one way for a practitioner to uncover his or her theories-in-use is to invite a trusted colleague to observe him or her in practice. Practitioners often hold different and incompatible theories-in-use (Argyris & Schön, 1992). Reflective practice invites practitioners to examine both their espoused theories and their theories-in-use; those locations where gaps exist between the two offer particularly rich opportunities for professional growth and development (Kinsella, 2001). As an example, in the audiology case study above, the practitioner recognized the need for flexibility within her theory of practice, as she came to see that every client and situation is unique, thus necessitating further development of her espoused theory of practice.

Benefits and Challenges

A number of potential benefits of reflective practice have been identified in the literature (Greenwood, 1998; Honor Society of Nursing, 2005;

Kinsella, 2000, 2001, 2007c; Schön, 1983, 1987), and are summarized below:

Reflective practice:

- fosters personal and professional development;
- is necessary for the development of professional expertise;
- encourages a holistic, individualized, and flexible approach to care;
- fosters the identification, description, and resolution of practical problems;
- enables the monitoring of increasing effectiveness over time;
- enables practitioners to explore and come to understand the nature and boundaries of their own role and that of other health professionals;
- validates practitioner knowledge and expertise generated through experience in practice;
- assists practitioners to better understand the conditions within which one practices, and, in particular, the barriers that might limit practitioners' therapeutic effectiveness;
- fosters an acceptance of professional responsibility;
- allows the generation of a knowledge base that is more comprehensive because it is directly related to what practitioners know about practice; and
- fosters practitioner engagement in reflective dialogue with team, client/patient, and family members, which may foster improved communication, health education, and interprofessional care.

While many potential benefits of reflective practice are highlighted, a number of challenges are also frequently identified. One of the biggest challenges is finding time for reflection. Reflection requires time, opportunity, and a supportive context. Many scholars have highlighted the significance of creating organizational cultures that support the reflective activities of health care practitioners as important for advancing professional learning (Argyris & Schön, 1992; Hatton & Smith, 1995; Kinsella, 2000; Mantzoukas & Jasper, 2004; McNamara, 1990).

In the midst of increasingly busy professional lives, frequently informed by what Stein (2002) has referred to as the 'cult of efficiency,' practitioners may find it difficult to find time for reflection or for reflective conversations with clients and colleagues. Busy workplaces often fail to promote cultures that support reflection, so that practitioners may feel that they are working against the grain when they try to integrate more time for reflection into their professional lives. In addition, the emphasis on evidence-based health care and outcome measures may inform a context that appears to value formal forms of scientific knowledge over the more practical forms of knowledge generated through reflection in and on particular case examples and professional practice, such that the knowledge generated from practice may not be recognized as legitimate. Nonetheless, a number of commentators have argued that reflective practice and evidence-based practice need not be seen as dichotomous (Kinsella, 2007a; Mantzoukas, 2007; Mantzoukas & Watkinson, 2008), and indeed that both are required for effective professional thinking (Bannigan & Moores, 2009).

Conclusion

In conclusion, despite the challenges of reflective practice, we have represented four practitioner/scholars whose lives have been changed through engagement with the theory of reflective practice and its application to our professional lives. In this chapter we've identified key concepts relevant to understanding and advancing reflective practice in allied health care disciplines, and offered case studies to illuminate these concepts through practical examples. While we do not see reflective practice as a panacea, we are committed to fostering reflective practice in allied health care (Caty, Kinsella, & Doyle, 2009; Jenkins, 2007, 2008; Kinsella, 2000, 2001, 2007a, 2007b, 2007c, 2009; Kinsella & Jenkins, 2007; Ng, 2009). We contend that this educational theory, one that recognizes the significance of practice experience as an important source of professional knowledge, has the potential to assist practitioners to navigate the indeterminate zones of practice and the frequently lamented gap between theory and practice. In addition, we propose that reflective practice has the capacity to enrich the lives and practices of health care practitioners, their clients, and the organizations in which they work. We advocate for workplaces in health care that foster a culture that facilitates and supports reflective practice.

REFERENCES

Argyris, C., & Schön, D. (1992). Theories in action. In Theory in practice: Increasing professional effectiveness (pp. 3–19). San Francisco: Jossey-Bass.
Bannigan, K., & Moore, A. (2009). A model of professional thinking: Integrating reflective practice and evidence based practice. Canadian Association of Occupational Therapy Journal, 5(76), 342–350.

Benner, P. (2001). From novice to expert: Excellence and power in clinical nursing practice [Commemorative edition]. Upper Saddle River, NJ: Prentice Hall.

Bolton, G. (2010). Reflective practice: Writing and professional development (3d ed.). London: Sage Publications.

Boud, D. (2001). Using journal writing to enhance reflective practice. New Directions for Adult and Continuing Education, 90, 9–17. doi: 10.1002/ace.16.

Brookfield, S. (1998). Critically reflective practice. The Journal of Continuing Education in the Health Professions, 18, 197–205.

Brookfield, S. (2000). The concept of critically reflective practice. In A. Wilson & E. Hayes (Eds.), Handbook of adult and continuing education (pp. 33–49). San Francisco: Jossey-Bass.

Caty, M.E., Kinsella, E.A., & Doyle, P. (2009). Linking the art of practice in head and neck cancer rehabilitation with the scientist's art of research: A case study on reflective practice. Canadian Journal of Speech-Language Pathology and Audiology, 33(4), 183–188.

Fenstermacher, G. (1988). The place of science and epistemology in Schön's conception of reflective practice. In P.P. Grimmett & G.L. Erickson (Eds), Reflection in teacher education (pp. 39–46). New York: Teachers College Press.

Greenwood, J. (1998). The role of reflection in single and double loop learning. Journal of Advanced Nursing Practice, 27(5), 1048–1053.

Greiner, A. C., & Knebel, E. (2003). Health professions education: A bridge to quality. Washington, DC: National Academy Press.

Grimmett, P.P., & Erickson, G.L. (Eds.). (1988). Reflection in teacher education (pp. 39–46). New York: Teachers College Press.

Hatton, N., & Smith, D. (1995). Reflection in teacher education: Towards definition and implementation. Teaching and Teacher Education, 11(1), 33–49.

Higgs, J., Richardson, B., & Dahlgren, M.A. (Eds.). (2004). Developing practice knowledge for health professionals. Oxford: Butterworth-Heinemann.

Honor Society of Nursing. (2005). The scholarship of reflective practice. In Honor Society of Nursing. Indianapolis, IN: Sigma Theta Tau International. http://www.nursingsociety.org/about/position_resource_papers.html.

Jenkins, K. (2007). Thinking differently about reflection. PHRED Focus Newsletter, 16(2), 1–3.

Jenkins, K. (2008). Pausing to reflect. PHRED Focus Newsletter, 17(1), 1–3.

Jenkins, K. (2011). Exploring public health nurse preceptors' experience of learning. (Unpublished master's thesis). University of Western Ontario, London, ON.

Johns, C. (2002). Guided reflection: Advancing practice. Oxford: Blackwell Science.

Kinsella, E.A. (2000). Professional development and reflective practice: Strategies for learning through professional experience. Ottawa: CAOT Publications.

Kinsella E.A. (2001). Reflections on reflective practice. Canadian Journal of Occupational Therapy, 68, 195–198.

Kinsella, E.A. (2007a). Technical rationality in Schön's reflective practice: Dichotomous or non-dualistic epistemological position. Nursing Philosophy, 8, 102–113.

Kinsella, E.A. (2007b). Embodied reflection and the epistemology of reflective practice. Journal of Philosophy of Education, 41(3), 395–409.

Kinsella, E.A. (2007c). Advanced topics in reflective practice. In A. Bossers et al. (Eds.), On-line preceptor education program: Preparing partners of learning in the field. www.preceptor.ca/index.html. University of Western Ontario, Faculty of Health Sciences & the Ontario Ministry of Health and Long Term Care.

Kinsella, E.A. (2009). Professional knowledge and the epistemology of reflective practice. Nursing Philosophy, 11 (1), 3–14.

Kinsella, E.A. & Jenkins, K. (2007). Fostering reflective practice. In A. Bossers, M.B. Bezzina, S. Hobson, A. Kinsella, A. MacPhail, S. Schurr, et al. (Eds.). On-line preceptor education program: Preparing partners of learning in the field. www.preceptor.ca/index.html. University of Western Ontario, Faculty of Health Sciences & The Ontario Ministry of Health and Long Term Care.

Kolb, D.A. (1984). Experiential learning: Experience as the source of learning and development. Englewood Cliffs, NJ: Prentice-Hall.

Mantzoukas, S. (2007). The evidence-based practice ideologies. Nursing Philosophy, 8(4), 244–255.

Mantzoukas, S., & Jasper, M.A. (2004). Reflective practice and daily ward reality: A covert power game. Journal of Clinical Nursing, 13(8), 925–933.

Mantzoukas, S., & Watkinson, S. (2008). Redescribing reflective practice and evidence-based practice discourses. International Journal of Nursing Practice, 14(2), 129–134.

McNamara, D. (1990). Research on teachers' thinking: Its contribution to educating student teachers to think critically. Journal of Education for Teaching, 16(2), 147–160.

Mezirow, J. (1990). Fostering critical reflection in adulthood: A guide to transformative and emancipatory learning. San Francisco: Jossey-Bass.

Moon, J. (1999). Reflection in learning and professional development: Theory and practice. London: Kogan Page.

228 Elizabeth Anne Kinsella et al.

Moon, J.A. (2004). A handbook of reflective and experiential learning: Theory and practice. New York: Routledge.

Ng, S. (2009). An introduction to reflective practice for audiologists. Audiology-Online. Published 29 June 2009 at http://www.audiologyonline.com/Articles/article_detail.asp?article_id=2248.

Polanyi, M. (1967). The tacit dimension. London: Routledge.

Ryle, G. (1949). The concept of mind. London: Hutchinson.

Sackett, D., Straus, S., Richardson, W., Rosenberg, W., & Haynes, R. (2000). Evidence-based medicine: How to practice and teach EBM (2d ed.). Edinburgh: Churchill Livingstone.

Schön, D. (1983). The reflective practitioner. New York: Basic Books.

Schön, D. (1987). Educating the reflective practitioner. San Francisco: Jossey-Bass.

Schön, D. (1992). The theory of inquiry: Dewey's legacy to education. Curriculum Inquiry, 22, 119-139.

Schön, D. (1994). Frame reflection: Towards the resolution of intractable policy controversies. New York: Basic Books.

Schön, D.A. (Ed.). (1991). The reflective turn. New York: Teachers College Press.

Stein, J. (2002). The cult of efficiency. Toronto: House of Anansi Press.

Van Manen, M. (1991). The tact of teaching: The meaning of pedagogical thoughtfulness. Albany: State University of New York Press.

White, S., Fook, J., & Gardner, F. (Eds.). (2006). Critical reflection in health and social care. Maidenhead, UK: Open University Press.

14 Physical Therapists as Educators in Clinical, Educational, and Community Settings

JOY HIGGS, FRANZISKA TREDE,
AND MEGAN SMITH

Achieving the goal of providing quality health care requires health professionals to determine what they understand by health and how they choose to implement health care. Increasingly in the twenty-first century health professionals, provider institutions, health professions, and clients are seeking collaborative forms of health care where clients participate in clinical decision-making and health care actions. In this environment health professionals are called upon to be educators, consultants, and partners rather than deliverers of intervention in the pursuit of illness remediation. In this context education has important roles to play as a practice approach, a therapeutic strategy, a means of quality assurance, and a communication medium with other professionals, clients, and their carers.

For physical therapists, health care has traditionally focused on enhancing movement and functional ability. In the twenty-first century physical therapists, like those in other professions, have encountered many challenges, including: expectations that their practice is strongly based on scientific evidence, demands from society for client-centred care, market forces, competition from other professions, external scrutiny in relation to both quality assurance and cost efficiency, and escalation of change in knowledge, practice, and technologies. Physical therapy as both a practice and political profession has responded to these influences in many ways, such as:

- the re-evaluation and diversification of the fields where physical therapists practice, with increasing employment beyond the traditional focus on acute health care institutions and private practice, to expand work in community health, health promotion, and consultancies;

- a trend in many countries towards graduate-entry education;
- an increasing emphasis on interprofessional collaboration; and
- a transition in the role of physical therapists, from care providers for individual clients to a greater emphasis on being health care educators, negotiators, collaborators, team leaders, and planners working with families, groups, communities, and society, as well as with individuals.

This chapter focuses on the role of physical therapy practitioners in clinical and community settings. We reflect on the place of the experiences and choices of physical therapy students and graduates that shape their approaches to practice and education. Starting with a definition of physical therapy today we explore learning and teaching in physical therapy education and in physical therapy practice. The notion of teaching in practice is also emphasized by Moseley (chapter 10) and Randall (chapter 11) in this book.

What Is Physical Therapy?

The World Confederation for Physical Therapy (WCPT, 2009) provides the following description:

> Physical therapy provides services to individuals and populations to develop, maintain and restore maximum movement and functional ability throughout the lifespan ... Functional movement is central to what it means to be healthy. Physical therapy is concerned with identifying and maximising quality of life and movement potential within the spheres of promotion, prevention, treatment/intervention, habilitation and rehabilitation. This encompasses physical, psychological, emotional, and social well being. Physical therapy involves the interaction between physical therapist, clients/clients, other health professionals, families, care givers, and communities in a process where movement potential is assessed and goals are agreed upon, using knowledge and skills unique to physical therapists. (p. 1)

Reasoning about teaching in practice has been identified as a specific and deliberate clinical reasoning strategy used by physical therapists (Edwards, Jones, Carr, Braunack-Mayer, & Jensen, 2004; Smith, Higgs, & Ellis 2007). These studies have identified that physical therapists across a range of settings integrate teaching with other aspects of their intervention. Teaching clients in physical therapy involves providing information to clients, instruction and guidance in activities, advice on courses of action, and explanations about movement problems and how they can be addressed.

Learning to be a Physical Therapist

Learning to be a physical therapist means learning to practise in this particular profession. Professional practice involves the capacity for doing, knowing, being, and becoming (Higgs & Titchen, 2001). A key to each of these processes is the active role of the practitioner (as well as the profession) in critically and creatively pursuing the delivery, education, and appraisal of quality practice:

> Our *doing* or practice role and intervention need to be individually tailored to the client's (or group's) needs, building on credible, defensible knowledge from our professional field and own experience. *Knowledge,* apart from being creatively used in practice situations, needs to be created through research, theory and experience to meet practice demands. Our *being,* the self we bring to professional practice, is a creative entity, meeting individual needs with individual solutions. Our *becoming* is a creative process and outcome, responding to our needs for growth and to our practice needs for development. (Higgs and Titchen, 2001, p. 5)

Becoming a Physical Therapist: Professional Socialization

Becoming a physical therapist is a continuing journey of professional socialization or acculturation (Higgs, Hummell, & Roe-Shaw, 2009). This process occurs through entry education, reflection, professional development, and engagement in professional work interactions. It involves learning about and becoming part of the culture and practice of the profession and the workplace; the individual develops the expected capabilities of the profession and a sense of professional identity and responsibility.

As a result of this acculturation, novice professionals develop their professional identity and gain knowledge of what it means to belong to the community of practice that is physiotherapy. They learn about professional codes of conduct, the roles and responsibilities of professionals, the profession-specific and generic capabilities of physiotherapists and health professionals, respectively, and the professional work context, including the goals, roles, and procedures of that system (Cant & Higgs, 1999).

Students become novice practitioners, and throughout their careers they continue to become more experienced and develop their professional identity through their own learning and choices. This learning involves coming to know about the expectations of their clients and their communities of practice; including workplace, professional, multidisciplinary, and socio-cultural communities. For example, you notice that people are not well educated about health issues and risk factors and they do not understand that their health is at least partly their responsibility. You may be very interested in addressing these issues and consider specializing in health promotion or health education aspects of physiotherapy.

Novice and experienced professionals make many choices, including: What type of practitioner do I want to be? Will my professional journey take me beyond clinical practice? What are the capabilities I need to be able to be and become the physiotherapist I wish to be? A key aspect of all of these choices is being a reflective and capable learner, and frequently the roles of physiotherapists as practitioners, educators, consultants, and leaders involve being a capable and facilitative teacher.

Exercise

Imagine you work with amputees and your goal is to help them to walk correctly (e.g., without hip circumduction); however, your amputee client is not interested in walking 'perfectly.' He wants to simply feel safe ambulating in his local area. Consider what you would do in these circumstances and go back and answer the questions in the paragraph above.

Interprofessional Practice and Education

Apart from discipline-specific education there is an international trend to involve health science students in interprofessional education and subsequently in interprofessional practice. The term 'interprofessional education' refers to education where students or members from two or more professions learn with, from, and about each other to improve collaboration and the quality of patient care (CAIPE, 2007). Elsewhere in this volume, Gastaldi and Hibbert, as well as Hibbert, Hunter, and Hibbert share this interest in interprofessional learning.

Learning in these contexts, both as students and graduate practitioners, provides a valuable means of preparing for professional practice, team work, and collaboration in health care. Such collaboration can be described as occurring in communities of practice. This term refers to the idea of communities or groups in a particular discipline or setting working together, setting norms and expectations of practice, and participating in the framing of that community. A key feature of these communities is that learning is embedded in practice rather than being a separate or optional activity (Higgs, Ajjawi, & Smith, 2009).

Cox (2005) refers to two key features of communities of practice: *situated negotiation of meaning* (i.e., locally and socially constructed knowledge), and *identity being central to learning*. What is important in communities of practice is that individuals learn and develop their professional identity by being part of the community. Yet this is not a passive development. Just as professionals have the privilege of professional autonomy and the responsibility for the actions they take in practise, they also have similar agency and responsibility for their own learning. Both involve individuals making choices and dealing with the outcomes of their actions, as well as responding to external influences. For each practitioner, his/her professional identity is shaped by these choices and situational drivers of the multiple communities they participate in. Beginning practitioners would need to develop an understanding of the communities of practice that are going to be shaping their practice. They could identify these communities by considering who they work with, who they learn from, and who they influence through their actions.

Exercise

Make a list of the various practice communities that you participate in. Identify for each of these: (a) What is your role, input, and authority? (b) What does that community expect of you? and (c) Who are the key players and what are their roles in that community?

Draw a cognitive map or diagram that shows how all of these factors interact, and then ask yourself the following questions:

- Am I satisfied with my role, identity, and contributions in these communities?
- How am I performing as a practitioner, learner, and educator in these situations?
- What learning or changes in my practice should I pursue to improve my practice?

Learning to be a Physical Therapist and Facilitate Learning in Others: The Place of Adult Learning

A central argument throughout this book is that adult learning provides a valuable framework for learning and teaching. Adult learning refers to how people learn, and is based on a number of assumptions, including the following, adapted from Knowles, Holton, and Swanson (1998, pp. 65–68).

Adult Learning Assumptions

• Adults become ready to learn the things they need to know and be able to do in order to cope effectively with their real-life situations. Therefore, these are the appropriate starting points for organizing adult learning activities.
• In contrast to children's subject-centred orientation to learning, adults are life-centred (or task/problem-centred) in their learning orientation. Therefore, the appropriate units for organizing adult learning are life situations, not subjects.
• Adults come into an educational activity with a greater volume and a different quality of experience than young people. Experience is the richest resource for adults' learning; therefore, the core methodology of adult education is the analysis of experience.
• Adults have a deep need to be self-directing; therefore, the role of the teacher is to engage in a process of mutual inquiry with them rather than transmit his or her knowledge to them and then evaluate their conformity to it.
• Individual differences among people increase with age; therefore, adult education must make optimal provision for differences in style, time, place, and pace of learning.
• Adults need to know why they need to learn something before undertaking to learn it.
• Adults have a self-concept of being responsible for their own decisions and lives.
• While adults are responsive to some external motivators (e.g., jobs), the most potent motivators are internal pressures (e.g., the desire for increased self-esteem; job satisfaction, such as success in client management; quality of life).

Conditions that facilitate adult learning have been examined by a number of scholars (Higgs, 2004). These conditions include Knowles's

(1980) principles of teaching, Knox's (1977) major generalizations about how teachers can facilitate adult learning, Bagnall's (1978) principles of effective adult learning, Schön's (1987) educating reflective practitioners, and Mezirow's (1981, 1985) Charter for Andragogy, based on the theories of Habermas (1971). Mezirow proposed that adult-learning teachers' decisions and actions need to give priority to the learner's developing autonomy. From the work of these authors it can be argued that adult-learning teachers have the role of creating key conditions for adult learning, including environmental conditions and conditions related to the decision-making and management strategies employed in the program (Table 14.1). In classrooms and practical work environments students commonly experience increasing autonomy during the successive years of their course. This would involve shifting from observation to guided practice to practising with peers in classroom practical sessions. In the clinical environment, junior students would be more heavily supervised and have fewer patients to treat. Senior students would ideally work largely independently following initial treatments under supervision, and be able to call upon advice from supervisors as needed.

Being a self-directed learner is central to adult learning and it is also a lifelong responsibility of professionals. Practitioners should be continually engaged in self-directed learning as they critique their knowledge, skills, and abilities and seek to enhance them. Self-directed learning embodies a number of key elements (Higgs, 2004). First, students bring different learning capabilities to the learning task (e.g., different levels of independence in learning). Second, they bring different experiences to learning, such as a variety of clinical education experiences, both positive and negative, success stories, and crises (for instance learning to cope with the death of a patient). Third, learning opportunities and teaching strategies can vary with differing levels of supervision, peer learning, pursuit of independent learning (e.g., on-line, through libraries, with colleagues), and modes of feedback. Fourth, self-directed learning involves learning outcomes such as learning how to be self-directed in learning, and learners taking responsibility for their learning outcomes rather than relying on teacher direction.

Reflection

How did you learn how to learn? Consider what you currently know and know how to do in relation to your practice – was this taught during your course or did you 'learn on the job'? As a professional of

Table 14.1. Adult Learning Behaviours and Conditions

Adult learning behaviours	Environmental conditions	Decision-making/ management factors
Empowered self-direction	Resource-rich environment	Goals are shared
Interaction with teacher, peers	Student-centred learning	Management of the learning program is shared
Active participation in learning	Freedom/autonomy	Mutual decision-making and planning occurs
Experiential learning	Individuality	Resource acquisition is shared
Self-correction	Emphasis on abilities and experience	Learners are actively involved in learning.
Reciprocal learning	High support and high challenge	Needs diagnosis, and evaluation
Self-criticality	Effective/appropriate group dynamics	Ongoing review by teacher and learners
Internal drive/ motivation	Interaction between learners	Learners pose questions and seek answers
Critical reflection	Motivation	Learners shape own learning context
Progressive mastery	Mutual respect and trust	Effective communication is pursued
Active seeking of meaning	Teacher support/ facilitation	Participation involves choice
Individual pacing	Learning via relevant experience	Facilitation is collaborative
Problem-posing and problem-solving	Praxis – integrating reflection, theory, practice, experience	Learners accept responsibility for learning
Enthusiasm for learning		Learners identify community goals and needs
Interdependence	Acceptance of learner as person	

Source: Terry & Higgs (1993)

today or tomorrow, what activities do you pursue to continue to learn and enhance your professional capabilities?

Learning to be a physical therapist is related to learning to educate others in physical therapy practice. For instance, beginning practitioners learning practice skills such as assisting clients with mobilization typically also have to learn how to educate clients and assistants about their role to ensure a positive outcome. Physical therapy practice requires the knowledge and actions of physical therapy to be shared and accessed by others: for example, during clinical education for novice practitioners, educating other disciplines about physical therapy practice, and client education. Adult learning principles are most suited to this purposeful, goal-oriented, and practice-focused form of education. When ownership, participation, and shared responsibility are required in educational situations then adult learning approaches are the choice of approach. However, if decisive action in a life-threatening situation is required, teacher direction is the choice of approach. Effective education requires a deep understanding of your own practice and the ability to unpack the hidden and implicit elements of the practice to make it accessible to others.

Exercise

Think of an aspect of physical therapy practice that you are very familiar with and are able to perform easily. How would you teach this practice to someone else? What are the important aspects of the practice? What are the obvious aspects of this process, and what are the hidden or implicit elements that you need to unpack to explain your practice to someone else?

Education Practice in Clinical and Community Settings

As a physical therapist you will engage in practice in a number of settings. For instance, the provision of physical therapy can occur in acute care health settings where physical therapy aids clients in the recovery from acute illness and in community-based settings where the emphasis may be on assisting clients to achieve optimal levels of function in their daily lives. In line with these diverse workplace and social contexts of practice, physical therapy can be provided to influence the health of individuals or populations. The choice of where physical therapists work can reflect individual preferences for specialty areas of physiotherapy practice such as acute care, rehabilitation, sports physical therapy, pediatrics, or geriatrics, but also reflects the prevailing politically based funding and priority health areas. The nature of education provided by physical therapists will be influenced by the type of physical therapist you want to be, the practice model you choose, the relationship you form with clients, and the contexts in which you practice.

Choosing What Type of Physical Therapist You Want to Be

Choosing what type of physical therapist you want to be is part of the process of becoming a professional. Here we are not thinking about what specialized area within physical therapy you choose to work, such as sports or geriatrics, but the values and interests that motivate you to become a physical therapist. The type of professional you want to become could range from becoming a technical expert giving advice, or a practical empathic collaborator with your clients, or a client advocate helping them achieve their health goals. The way we learn and practise is influenced by what we are interested in, what we want to listen to, and what we want to engage with (Trede & Higgs, 2009). Becoming a physical therapist is therefore also about observing, reflecting, and judging critically how others think, act, and conduct themselves as physical therapists. For example, when learning to practise in an environment with many experienced health professionals there are many exemplars of practice for new practitioners to observe and learn from. As well as observing, beginning practitioners need to critically judge what they see, and reflect upon decisions they are making about the way that they will practise. There will be colleagues you are working with who display characteristics, attitudes, and expertise that you admire and there will be other colleagues who display characteristics and attitudes that you might find undesirable.

Reflection

Think about three physical therapists whom you consider being your role models. Write down what it is about these people that you respect and admire. Include their characteristics, approaches to practice, communication style, reasoning and reflecting, attitudes towards clients, carers, and colleagues. Reflect upon how closely your behaviour and practice approach resembles these characteristics and what actions or learning you would need to pursue to become more like your role models.

Choosing a Practice Model and the Type of Educator You Will Be

Health care practice models have been categorized into three broad categories: biomedical, psychosocial, and emancipatory (Szasz & Hollender, 1956; Trede & Higgs, 2009). These three categories are located in three different theoretical and philosophical paradigms. Habermas (1971), a prominent philosopher, claimed that knowledge and practice is influenced by the questions that are asked and not asked, by what is perceived as important and not important. According to Habermas, the way professionals think, make decisions, educate clients, and act, in short how they make sense of their practice, is based on professional values and interests. These values and interests might be unconsciously or consciously chosen but they nevertheless shape physical therapists' choice of practice model. The purpose and benefit of consciously choosing a practice model enables (novice) physical therapists to become active participants in the future direction of their professional development and their profession. It also equips physical therapists with skills to question taken-for-granted and unreflected ways of practising, and liberates them to transform their practice to be highly appropriate and effective in their ever-changing work and client contexts. Table 14.2 illustrates three broad practice models and their related differences to educational approaches and teaching methods.

We argue that it is important to draw out hidden interests behind human interactions and systems. Biomedical interests focus on reducing deficits and symptoms with the aim of controlling and predicting; these are technical interests in provider-determined best practice settings. An example would be physical therapists selecting interventions that aim to improve the range of motion of a joint and using these with the client. Practical interests help clients cope and adjust to current structures and norms with the aim of working together. Emancipatory interests aim to facilitate autonomy, self-determination, and mature negotiated practice.

Educating Clients to Become Informed and Collaborative Decision-makers

Educating clients is a complex task that goes beyond telling clients medical facts. Education for informed and collaborative decision-making involves finding out what clients already know and meaningfully filling in knowledge gaps, demystifying or even challenging unreflected assumptions about movement, functional disability, and pain, and their treatment approaches; identifying what is most important to clients; negotiating common ground and shared goals; and supporting ongoing learning. It also involves ascertaining the client's capacity for informed decision-making and when others (e.g., carers and health professionals)

Table 14.2. Three Practice Models and Their Related Educational Approaches

Practice model	Biomedical	Psychosocial	Emancipatory
	Health is located in the physical world	Health is located in the social world	Health is located in the political world
	Practice knowledge is based on empirical data	Practice knowledge comprises propositional, personal, and professional craft knowledges	Practice knowledge is based on democratic and social justice values; political aspects are also included
	Physical aspects of clients are the focus of interest and concern	Physical, mental, and spiritual aspects of clients are of interest and concern	Socio-cultural and historical aspects of clients and communities are of interest and concern
	Clinician-client relationships reflect differential expert-lay relationships	Clinician-client relationships acknowledge expertise of both parties	Clinician-client relationships are democratic and mutually respectful
	Evidence has an outcome-driven, quantitative connotation	Evidence has a contextual, process-driven connotation	Evidence has an emancipatory connotation
Educational approach	Didactic	Experiential	Critical
	Telling clients what is best for them	Two-way flow of information	Identifying what clients already know and helping them learn what they need to know to achieve their health goal
	Emphasising contents and instructions	Exploring best solution within context	Emphasizing transparent and critical dialogues
	Propositional knowledge represents *the* 'truth'	Accepting multiple realities	
Teaching methods	Structured Active-passive Objective	Informal Experiential Reflective	Informal Participatory Critically reflective

need to assist with or make decisions for clients who do not have this capacity. For instance, in circumstances where an unconscious client is admitted to emergency following a motor vehicle accident, a physician might be required to make intervention decisions on the client's behalf. The aim of client (and carer) education is to engage clients (and carers) in making relevant and realistic decisions that have positive and sustainable outcomes. Making decisions *with* and not *for* clients is tailored to clients' interests and capacities and ensures shared responsibility in the sustained pursuit of agreed decisions. Shared decisions are more likely to embrace biomedical, psychosocial, and empowering aspects of health.

Health care systems and the roles of clinicians and clients are constantly being transformed. Communicating with and educating clients is now seen as being just as important as treating clients (NSW Health, 2005). Advances in medical technology, as well as the inability to find cures for certain diseases such as cancer and HIV/AIDS in the short-term, make educating clients for self-management a prime aspect of providing care. Further, clients (and carers) want to be involved and actively collaborate in their health management. For example, clients who are encouraged to talk about medication side effects or pain resulting from prescribed exercises are more likely to learn and improve medication or exercise regimens than clients who feel their experiences do not count. Collaboration means that the clients' (and carers) perspectives are valued, listened to, and integrated into the decision-making process just as the professionals' perspectives are. Such collaboration is based on mutual respect. It blends the scientific with the social world and thus humanizes the decision-making process.

Collaborative approaches to clinical decision-making raises issues of professional authority and educational roles. Physical therapists who engage in collaboration are willing to share responsibility and are responding to their clients' priorities. Collaboration does not mean allowing clients to raise their concerns, expectations, and hopes, to then have them ignored. Such an approach is not collaborative but asserts professional authority over clients and at worst is patronizing. However, it is important to note that collaborative approaches do not imply that physical therapists are giving up their professional expertise or that they are just providing whatever the client requests. It does imply that such therapists are critically reflecting on what it means to practise physical therapy in the twenty-first century, and responding by transforming their practice to include client education approaches that promise sustainable, culturally appropriate, and effective outcomes for their clients.

Case Example:

A male physical therapist student came to mobilize a Turkish woman on her first day after surgery. Initially she was smiling, but when the therapist mentioned mobilization the client became anxious and refused to get out of bed. The physical therapist assumed that the reason for refusing was cultural. He went to ask his supervisor for help. Surprisingly, the patient now mobilized without resistance. During the walk she told the two therapists that at a previous mobilization she had a fall, which made her anxious to mobilize with one person only. The student learned from this experience not to interpret client behaviours based on unreflected and unchecked assumptions.

Exercise

Write your honest, self-appraisal responses to the following questions:

- Do I think it is a good idea to give clients an opportunity to tell their story and ask questions or question my advice?
- What are my strengths in helping clients learn?
- As a therapist what teaching aspects would I like to strengthen in my practice?

Choosing a View of Health

Reflection

Rank the following people from healthiest to least healthy:

- Professional rugby player with a left knee reconstruction
- Director of a law firm who is a chain-smoker
- University professor living with depression
- Single mother with breast cancer
- Landscape gardener who is unemployed
- A person with a chronic disability who considers she has an effective self- management approach

This ranking exercise helps us to reflect upon what is meant by health. Health means different things to different people. The exercise helps us think about the way health is understood and what people value most about health. Values about health shape the way health professionals practice and the approaches they adopt to educate clients. Values about health and well-being shape the way people use their bodies and live their lives.

If health is viewed in a biomedical sense as the opposite of being ill, as an absence of pathology, then physical therapists could be seen as scientists who intervene by providing therapy to people with movement-related dysfunctions. Education in this context is probably limited to teaching clients how to comply with prescribed treatments. On the other hand, health can be viewed as capabilities, defined as follows:

> Health is ... seen as a resource for everyday life, not the objective of living. Health is a positive concept emphasizing social and personal resources, as well as physical capacities. (WHO, 1986, p. 1)
>
> Health potential can be best achieved when clients' personal integrity remains intact, their quality of life is enhanced, and when they gain an improved sense of control over their health with long-term sustainability wherever possible. (Trede & Higgs, 2003, p. 67)

In this view of health we are faced with a different set of questions and choices. Our clients may be people who are ill and being cared for in hospital; they may be disabled and receiving therapy in rehabilitation centres; they may be people accessing community health services; or they may be well and searching for improved health, fitness, and well-being. As discussed above, practitioners' practice models are influenced by many things; this includes their view of health. A key consequence of having a wellness practice model is giving emphasis to the role of physical therapists as educators. Here education includes sharing professional knowledge to help clients make informed choices, presenting self-treatment options, explaining the strengths and limitations of self-management or treatment options that clients find for themselves on the Web, and teaching families how to be players in treatment support options. For example, physical therapists working with children with disabilities in an early intervention setting would engage in a model of education that emphasizes collaboration with families about optimal courses of intervention.

Factors Influencing These Choices

Smith, Higgs, and Ellis (2007) identified that physical therapy decision-making was shaped by the context in which it occurred. This shaping of decision-making extended to the use of teaching as an intervention and interaction strategy. The physical therapists in this study varied their approach to education depending upon the time available, the acuteness of the client's illness, the client's cognitive state and the duration of the relationship they were forming with clients. Where clients were experiencing chronic illnesses and a long-term relationship was involved, greater emphasis was given to education as a strategy. This contrasted with short duration interventions where teaching was directed more towards didactic approaches. That is, physical therapists are likely to vary their approach to teaching clients according to contextual demands.

Exercise

Consider the circumstances of your practice: How do the contextual influences present in your work shape your approach to teaching? How are you influenced by the time and resources available or the actions of colleagues? What value is placed on teaching as an intervention strategy?

Conclusion

Physical therapy practice in health care is intimately entwined with educational practice. This chapter has described the embedded nature of teaching in the reasoning processes and interventions of physical therapists. We have argued that learning to educate in physical therapy is grounded in the process of learning to be a physical therapist. To educate others requires a deep understanding of our own practices and the values and knowledge that underpins these practices. The nature of education in physical therapy is most closely aligned with the conditions and behaviours of adult education. Although teaching practices in clinical and community settings has been the subject of some research, there is considerable scope to more deeply explore teaching practices, in particular the models of teaching that are employed, and how these models align with client needs and expectations of education for their health.

REFERENCES

Bagnall, R.G. (1978). Principles of adult education in the design and management of instruction. *Australian Journal of Adult Education, 28,* 19–27.

Cant, R., & Higgs, J. (1999). Professional socialisation. In J. Higgs & H. Edwards (Eds.), *Educating beginning practitioners: Challenges for health professional education* (pp. 46–51). Oxford: Butterworth-Heinemann.

CAIPE (Centre for the Advancement of Interprofessional Education). (2007). Definition of interprofessional education. Retrieved 20 July 2007 from www. caipe.org.uk.

Cox, A. (2005). What are communities of practice? A comparative review of four seminal works. *Journal of Information Science, 31*(6):527–540.

Edwards, I., Jones, M., Carr, J., Braunack-Mayer, A., & Jensen, G. (2004). Clinical reasoning strategies in physical therapy. *Physical Therapy, 84*(4), 312–335.

Habermas, J. (1971). *Knowledge and human interests.* Boston: Beacon Press.

Higgs, J. (2004). Educational theory and principles related to learning clinical reasoning. In M.A. Jones & D.A. Rivett (Eds.), *Clinical reasoning for manual therapists* (pp. 379–402). Edinburgh: Butterworth Heinemann.

Higgs, J., Ajjawi, R., & Smith, M. (2009). Working and learning in communities of practice. In J. Higgs, M. Smith, G. Webb, M. Skinner, & A. Croker (Eds.), *Contexts of physiotherapy practice* (pp. 117–127). Melbourne: Elsevier Australia.

Higgs, J., Hummell, J., & Roe-Shaw, M. (2009). Becoming a member of a health profession: A journey of socialisation. In J. Higgs, M. Smith, G. Webb, M. Skinner, & A. Croker (Eds.), *Contexts of physiotherapy practice* (pp. 58–71). Melbourne: Elsevier Australia.

Higgs, J., & Titchen, A. (2001). Framing professional practice: Knowing and doing in context. In J. Higgs & A. Titchen (Eds.), *Professional practice in health, education and the creative arts* (pp. 3–5). Oxford: Blackwell Science.

Knowles, M.S. (1980). *The modern practice of adult education – from pedagogy to andragogy.* New York: Adult Education Company.

Knowles, M.S., Holton, E.F., & Swanson, R.A. (1998). *The adult learner* (5th ed.). Woburn, MA: Butterworth-Heinemann.

Knox, A.B. (1977). *Adult development and learning.* San Francisco: Jossey-Bass.

Mezirow, J. (1981). A critical theory of adult learning and education. *Adult Education, 32,* 3–24.

Mezirow, J. (1985). Concept and action in adult education. *Adult Education Quarterly, 35,* 142–151.

NSW Health. (2005). *Patient Safety and Clinical Quality Program: First Report of Incident Management in the NSW Public Health Care System 2003–2004.* Publication SHPN (QBS) 040262. Sydney: NSW Department of Health.

Schön, D.A. (1987). *Educating the reflective practitioner: Towards a new design for teaching and learning in professions.* San Francisco: Jossey-Bass.

Smith, M., Higgs, J., & Ellis, E. (2007). Physiotherapy decision-making in acute cardiorespiratory care is influenced by factors related to the physiotherapist and the nature and context of the decision: A qualitative study. *Australian Journal of Physiotherapy, 53*(4), 261–267.

Szasz, T.S., & Hollender, M.H. (1956). A contribution to the philosophy of medicine. *Archives of Internal Medicine, 97*, 585–592.

Terry, W., & Higgs, J. (1993). Educational programmes to develop clinical reasoning skills. *Australian Journal of Physiotherapy, 39*(1), 47–51.

Trede, F., & Higgs, J. (2003). Reframing the clinician's role in collaborative clinical decision-making: Rethinking practice knowledge and the notion of clinician-client relationships. *Learning in Health and Social Care, 2*(2), 66–73.

Trede, F., & Higgs, J. (2009). Models and philosophy of practice. In J. Higgs, M. Smith, G. Webb, M. Skinner, & A. Croker (Eds.), *Contexts of physiotherapy practice* (pp. 90–101). Melbourne: Elsevier Australia.

WCPT. (2009). Position statement: Description of physical therapy. World Confederation for Physical Therapy. Retrieved 20 September 2009 from http://www.wcpt.org/sites/wcpt.org/files/files/WCPT_Description_of_ Physical_Therapy-Sep07-Rev_2.pdf.

WHO. (1986). *Ottawa Charter of Health Promotion*. Geneva: World Health Organization.

15 Interprofessional Education for Sports' Health Care Teams: Using the CanMEDs Competencies' Framework

BRIAN GASTALDI AND KATHRYN HIBBERT

According to Statistics Canada (1994), 'The continuous and effective upgrading of Canada's human resources has become an essential condition of ensuring long term growth and success in the global economy. In the coming years, the changing demands of the workforce will put a lot of pressure on Canadian workers. Traditional jobs, with work patterns and skills that remain stable over the worker's entire career, are disappearing (pp. 5–6).

Echoes of this call continue to be heard today (CHSRF, 2006; Government of Ontario, 2005; Suter & Deutschlander, 2010; WHO, 2009). Providing quality health care for sports' participants and education for the professionals involved has become a costly and complex endeavour for many nations, including Canada. The creation of interprofessional sports' health care teams is one response that has emerged in an attempt to simultaneously address economic and educational challenges. Sports' health care teams can include a diverse collection of affiliated professionals such as physicians, chiropractors, massage therapists, physical therapists, athletic therapists, kinesiologists, and psychologists. In many ways, the practice of working collaboratively in the care and treatment of athletes has emerged as a natural extension of the sport team concept. In this chapter, we consider a model of continuing professional education (CPE) for sports' health care teams that translates into improved patient education and care, as it has with other professions that have adopted a core competencies model. Verma, Broers, Paterson, Schroder, Medves, and Morrison (2009), for instance, show how this model has been applied to medical radiation technology, social work, pharmacy, and psychology.

We begin by reviewing a physical therapy encounter using the fictional case of an elite hockey player named Allan. Allan's case may be instructive for both undergraduate and continuing professional education learners and instructors in all of the affiliated professions serving on a sports' health care team. Further, we offer suggestions for how we might improve interprofessional education by leveraging the highly successful 'CanMEDs' framework, developed by the Royal College of Physicians and Surgeons as a model for advanced practitioner training. We envision incorporating the framework into professional education for sports' health care workers drawing on principles of interprofessional education: 'Interprofessional Education [IPE] is about health professional program students learning how to practice together effectively in collaborative teams, where all members of teams are respected for their knowledge and skills ... [IPE] requires four levels of active learning: (a) gaining the knowledge needed about each other's disciplines to work together; (b) gaining experience working through case studies, as a collaborative team; (c) gaining collaborative team practice in simulated situations; and (d) gaining clinical experience with actual patients (clients) as a collaborative team' (Orchard, 2009, n.p.).

The fluidity of the four levels of active learning suggests possibilities to integrate IPE instruction from initial professional education through to continuing professional education experiences. This concern for interprofessional learning is shared by Higgs, Trede, and Smith in chapter 14 in this book, as well as in Hibbert, Hunter, and Hibbert in chapter 16.

The Role of an Interprofessional Sports Health Care Team

According to Hall and Weaver (2001), 'The [interprofessional] team refers to a team whose members work together closely and communicate frequently to optimize care for the patient. The team is organized around solving a common set of problems (as opposed to being organized around a single physician) ... Each member of the team contributes his/her knowledge and skill set to augment and support the others' contributions' (p. 868).

Importantly, affiliated members of the team each bring discipline-specific knowledge and skills to the health and welfare of the injured athlete. Each of the professions is responsible not only for the care of the patient, but also for observing the standards and conduct guidelines that regulate their practice. As Engel (1994) has noted, collaboration amongst a diverse group of professionals with different and sometimes competing discourses and procedures requires a sophisticated level of communication and negotiation skills. He therefore recommends that 'applicable competences should thus be developed quite deliberately throughout every undergraduate or basic training programme' (p. 72). While this early learning may serve to orient emerging professionals to the notion of teamwork, and familiarize them with the similarities and differences in their roles, ongoing learning will be necessary to soften the boundaries and rivalries that too often exist between professions. To situate the reader, we use the case of 'Allan' to describe a typical patient encounter with the health care system in Ontario, Canada.

The Case of 'Allan'

Allan is an 18-year-old accomplished hockey player who realizes that despite being a good junior hockey player, he is unlikely to be drafted by a professional hockey team. His ambition is to get a scholarship to play university hockey. He has had several minor injuries thus far in his career, but all have been resolved with a conservative (non-surgical) intervention. While playing in a pick-up softball game, he twists his left knee. He believes he felt something 'pop' in the knee, and over the course of the night the knee becomes significantly swollen.

Allan's father is able to prevail upon the family physician, who has attended Allan for most of his childhood and adolescent life, to see his son on an emergency basis early the following afternoon. During the appointment, the family physician listens to Allan's history of the injury, does a brief examination of his knee, and informs him that he has likely 'bruised' the knee, and that it should settle down in a matter of a few days. The family physician does not feel an X-ray series is warranted.

Allan returns home and relates to his parents what his family physician has said about the injury and its likely course. But Allan has an uneasy feeling about the extent of his knee injury, and after two days, in which it had shown no improvement, elects to visit the office of a physiotherapist, Patrick, from whom he has sought treatment for his previous injuries. Allan recalls that Patrick was thorough in his assessment of each of the injuries, offered effective clinical care which always included a good remedial exercise program, and helped guide Allan to a complete functional recovery and return to full activity.

Patrick is an experienced physiotherapist, having practiced for over 25 years. He has achieved advanced certification in both orthopedic and sport physiotherapy specialties. He currently conducts a small private practice, but for 20 of his years in practice, Patrick worked as a senior physiotherapist in one of the largest and best-known sport medicine clinics in Canada. He has extensive training in the assessment of injured and post-surgical knee injuries, their treatment, and graded rehabilitation.

Patrick maintains close professional and personal ties with the primary care physicians and orthopedic surgeons with whom he had worked for many years at the Sport Medicine Clinic. His work is highly regarded.

At the appointment, Patrick takes a thorough history of Allan's injury mechanism, and conducts a thorough physical examination of the knee. Based on this assessment, Patrick concludes that Allan has, in fact, torn the medial meniscus (cartilage) in his left knee. Patrick shares his findings with Allan, and asks his permission to tell his parents. Allan is a bit reluctant at first, because he had been advised by his father to avoid physical activities and sports that might lead to injury, and thus possibly derail his aspirations to play intercollegiate hockey. Patrick reasons with Allan, recalling that Allan's parents have always been supportive of Allan's athletic pursuits and have been there to help him through his other injuries. Patrick suggests that Allan be assessed by a primary care physician at the Sport Medicine Clinic, and from there, if appropriate, obtain a referral to an orthopedic consultant.

Patrick arranges for Allan to see Dr Tse, a primary care physician at the clinic, that afternoon. Dr Tse agrees with Patrick's findings and concludes, like Patrick, that the meniscus is likely torn, and is in need of a surgical repair – a procedure that, for a young man, allows him to have an excellent recovery and a reduced likelihood of early joint breakdown (shortly) after the surgery. Dr Tse arranges an orthopedic consultation with Dr Williams, who orders an M.R.I. of Allan's knee, which demonstrates definitively the meniscal tear. Dr Williams further suggests that a surgical repair is the best short- and long-term option, and is able to fit Allan into a cancellation early the following week. Allan agrees with the plan, and returns to Patrick's office to confirm the initial suspicion and the plan for a surgical intervention. He also asks Patrick to conduct his post-operative treatment and rehabilitation once the surgeon gives the go-ahead. Patrick agrees, and having overseen many such treatment interventions, is confident he can help Allan recover his full function.

Discussion of the Case

Allan's experience follows a typical trajectory of a patient encounter with the health care system and offers the reader a window into where the patient education typically occurs. An injury of this type frequently leads a patient to visit a primary health care physician on an emergency basis. Preliminary assessment is done to rule out the presence of a fracture. If either X-ray, or, in this case, a physical assessment does not indicate a fracture, the assumption is that the injury involves only the soft tissue and a prescription of rest and ice are usually prescribed. Allan's concern for his full recovery led him to seek advice from a physiotherapist with whom he had a trusting relationship and previous experience managing recovery from injury. Research has shown that the 'patient's perception of control over the problem and ability to cope are considered important indicators of a successful outcome' (Thomeé, Wahrborg, Borjesson, Thomee, Eriksson, & Karlsson, 2007, p. 486).

Patient education has been a part of physiotherapists' roles and responsibilities for decades. Indeed, patient education forms a part of nearly all physiotherapist-patient encounters, suggesting that 'patients can neither effectively participate in their treatment nor accept responsibility for their own care if they are not informed about what is wrong with them' (Sluijs, 1991, p. 562). However, many physiotherapists are reluctant to assert themselves in a situation where they believe a problem has been either misdiagnosed or under-diagnosed, thereby putting the patient at risk for a compromised quality of life. In this case, Patrick had the advanced training, experience, and close professional and personal relationship to a team of specialists that had developed over time. The working relationship that had developed between them was one of mutual trust and respect for the knowledge that each brought to the care and treatment of the patient.

This is not currently the case for many patients seeking treatment for an injury. In the existing health care model, the primary care physician often serves as the gatekeeper to care. It is typically only the primary care physician who is able to refer a patient to a specialist such as an orthopedic surgeon, or for follow-up care and treatment by an affiliated health care team member, such as a physiotherapist. In this model, care operates around the expertise and communication of the primary care physician. We wonder, what might a model look like if it centred on the type of injury encountered, and a flow of communication that includes the knowledge and expertise of other members of a sports' health care team in establishing the diagnosis and treatment plan. Hall and Weaver (2001) describe this process as 'role blurring,' suggesting that 'in teamwork, members should possess areas of overlapping competencies and share responsibilities depending on the model of practice.' However, they have observed that 'problems arise when role blurring is not handled well. Some team members may not realize the others' potential contribution to patient care, and will underutilize their expertise' (p. 871). In our experience working within interprofessional educational contexts, participants mutual lack of understanding of the knowledge and skills each has to bring to the patient encounter suggests a need for improved education.

In this case, Patrick informed Allan what was amiss with his knee, and offered a prognosis as to how it should be managed. He then continued the communication by conveying his findings and conclusions to the family physician, despite the fact that they differed from the physician's diagnosis: that it was just a 'bruised' knee that will get better with time. He also informed Allan's parents of his prognosis, helping them to realize that this was a manageable injury, from which Allan should have a full functional recovery. Further, he related his findings to the primary care physician, Dr Tse, proposing the need for an orthopedic referral, which Dr Tse arranged. Finally, he discussed his findings with the orthopedic consultant, as well as his perceived need for early management of the injury to avoid further morbidity from the injury. A number of competencies demonstrated through this health care encounter suggest promising possibilities for improving interprofessional education for sports' health care teams.

Building on an Existing Model: The CanMEDs' Competencies

Hall and Weaver (2001) have suggested that 'traditionally it is the physician who is responsible for prescribing the contribution other disciplines could make and for coordination of services. Team members work in parallel to each other and direct [interprofessional] communication is minimal except through the physician in charge' (p. 868). We considered what might happen if we reconceptualized the traditional model in ways that acknowledge the broader competencies of the sports' health care team. The approach to adopting a competencies' framework is one that has recently been taken up in a 'National Interprofessional Competency Framework' (2010) building on the successful CANMEDs framework already in use, for example, in medicine and occupational therapy.

The Royal College of Physicians and Surgeons of Canada defines the national standards for the education, assessment, and certification of medical and surgical specialists. The 1996 standards, *Skills for the New Millennium* (Frank et al., 1996), were rewritten as the *CanMEDs 2005 Physician Competency Framework*, 'updated for the nature of contemporary medicine, and its wording revised for greater clarity and utility' (Frank, 2005, p. 5). The revised document is a 'competency-based framework that describes the principal generic abilities of physicians oriented to optimal health and health care outcomes' (p. 5). The CanMEDs' framework has 'influenced or has been adopted in at least 17 jurisdictions around the world. It has also been used in the frameworks of at least 8 health professions' (Frank, 2008, p. 405). The seven CanMEDs' competencies include Medical Expert, Professional, Communicator, Collaborator, Manager, Health Advocate, and Scholar. These competencies are global in their scope and nature, and their universal application in international contexts is, in part, what has led other countries to embrace them.

Given its success, we propose that the CanMEDs' framework could be useful in developing interprofessional educational opportunities for sports' health care teams. As we reviewed the case of Allan, we were struck by how many of the physician competencies overlap with the role assumed by the physiotherapist, Patrick. Drawing on his significant experience and expertise in sports injury care, Patrick demonstrated the Manager role by initiating a consultation with a primary care physician in the sports medicine field along with recommendations for referral to an orthopedic surgeon. He demonstrated the Health Advocate role through carefully explaining his findings to both the patient and the patient's parents, along with a plan for rehabilitation to achieve the ultimate goal that he knew Allan was seeking: that of returning to a level of wellness to compete for a sports scholarship at the university level. Blurred across these actions are the roles of Communicator, Collaborator and Professional. Patrick's actions stem from the core competency, in this case Physiotherapy Expert, and, by sharing this case with a broader audience as a potential source for further learning and discussion, he has demonstrated the role of Scholar.

In this brief example, it seems not only plausible but promising to engage others in the sports' health professions education in interprofessional learning that centre on the CanMEDs' competencies. For example, in the case of Allan we suggest that readers do the following:

- Outline the key points of Allan's encounter with the health care system, and note any opportunities for professional education, and which knowledge, skill, or competency could be improved.
- Track the decision-making process of the parties: the family doctor, the physiotherapist, the patient, the primary care physician at the clinic, and the orthopedic surgeon. Consider what motivated their decision, what the outcome of their decision was, and what type of feedback they received about the outcome of their decision.

One of the challenges of implementing interprofessional learning has been finding the resources to both educate and implement teams of people across the professions. Building upon an existing model expected of the physician – already at the core of the current patient care model – may present achievable opportunities to bring members of the health care team together around a common focus. For example, raising awareness about the role that communication can play as various professionals involved in the health care team interact around the patient encounter can serve, not only to develop communication skills but also to help all members of the team come to appreciate the various skills and abilities that each has to offer to the overall plan for care. Understanding and learning to communicate effectively promises to ensure that appropriate professional involvement is secured early, potentially reducing the possibility of misdiagnosis or under-diagnosis. Once allied professionals better understand the knowledge and skills that each bring to a patient encounter, it is more likely that a shift towards organizing care based on the type of injury may be possible. Timely cost effective use of resources is another likely outcome that serves both the patient and the health care system.

Moving Forward

According to Hall and Weaver (2001), 'the concept of [interprofessional] teamwork did not originate in the university health sciences programs, but was formulated by front-line practitioners facing the complexities of patient care ... extreme pressures on the university system demand flexibility and responsiveness from the educational process' (p. 873).

It would appear that such extreme pressures are facing the health care system in a chronic way, and that these pressures demand innovative thinking about what it means to provide 'relevant, equitable, and sustainable access to health knowledge' (UNESCO, 1997, p. 5) If we agree that the development of interprofessional health care teams will play an increasing role in our health care response, we need to conceptualize new ways of engaging in the health care encounter with patients, their families, and the allied professionals who will play a role. Patrick recognized that his experience participating in a large sports' medicine clinic had provided him with multiple and rich forms of interprofessional learning informally in the work environment. For example, ongoing conversations permitted a sharing of expertise flowing in both directions allowed physiotherapists to better understand the needs of the orthopedic surgeons, and allowed surgeons to better understand the skills and knowledge physiotherapists contribute to both the nature of the injury and the follow-up care.

Not all physiotherapists will be situated in such a well organized learning environment. However, structured learning exists across all of the health and medical professions and it would seem prudent to build upon the existing infrastructure to provide continuing professional education in the workplace. For example, established clinical rounds are often attended by staff across multiple professions. It seems plausible that such rounds could be organized to foster interprofessional education by including presentations that focused on a case involving a sports' injury could be led by a physiotherapist. This reconceptualization suggests that we shift the centre of the encounter away from its current path that requires the general practitioner (i.e., family physician or emergency room physician) to carry the burden of gatekeeper in contexts that may well exist beyond the scope of their expertise and experience. Instead, teams that revolve around particular types of injury or illness can broaden the scope for intervention, diagnosis, and care. Shifting the focus in this way allows multiple ideas surrounding an injury to be considered. Hall and Weaver (2001) have suggested that 'idea dominance means that a clear and recognizable idea must serve as a focus for teamwork, rather than the traditional focus of each member's domain of care. This would place the patient at the centre of the team's focus. In addition, idea dominance emphasizes that the team members must be able to recognize their success and achievements in pursuing their goals' (p. 869).

Instructors responsible for initial and continuing education in the allied professions that comprise sports' health care teams might consider the following questions:

- How might the case of Allan provide an authentic example in which learners across professions (new and continuing) engage in collaborative dialogue in ways that foster application of knowledge?
- In what ways does an interprofessional case open up possibilities for creative and critical thinking skills?
- In what ways might sharing responsibility for learning (direction, leadership, and content) engage learners more actively?
- In what ways might drawing on authentic examples from practice bring awareness to opportunities for improved education?
- What might the encounter of Allan look like if told from the perspective of the athlete? The orthopedic surgeon? The family doctor?

- In what ways might developing shared competencies in the context of a shared practice trigger opportunities for improved communication across all team members (e.g., opportunities for explanation of decisions, concerns about treatment, recognition, and respect for diverse skills and knowledge)?
- How might each member of the team be responsible for bringing and leading a case example to target one of the competencies?

Returning to the case of Allan, there are a few issues and cautions that apply. First, it is widely recognized in all of the health professional/medical education settings that the current curriculum that prepares them for practice is already crowded. Adding to it will only increase the pressure to cover these topics in superficial ways. Second, the physiotherapist in this case, Patrick, is an experienced professional with advanced training, working primarily in the specialized field of sports' medicine. Although he is currently in private practice, he spent many years working collaboratively with allied professionals in a large sports medicine clinic. The conditions to develop the competencies across the professions were ripe in this informal learning context. Close collaboration allowed the skills and abilities of various professionals to be visible, and offered numerous opportunities for communication and the development of a shared understanding of types of injury, treatment options, and outcomes over time. The likelihood of professional consultation leading to a shared diagnosis and prognosis increases in this scenario, thus reducing the chance that a patient would receive conflicting conclusions about an injury and inappropriate course of action such as Allan experienced. The development of professional rapport, collaboration, and credibility in the workplace makes it more likely that interprofessional training based on a framework such as CanMEDs competencies (designed to be integrated into medical curriculum at the undergraduate, postgraduate, and continuing medical education levels) would succeed. Such an approach could leverage the existing structures of time and space in ways that promise to ultimately improve patient care. Costs for developing professional education at all levels on a model like this could be shared, thus lightening the load for any single professional organization both in terms of developing a program and implementing it. The real potential lies in the pre-service and continuing interprofessional education opportunities that bring together professionals who share a common goal. Care for elite athletes, like many patients, typically involves interactions with a number of health care professionals who each play a distinct role in diagnosis, treatment, patient education, and follow-up. The concept of interprofessional education reflects the reality of professional practice. All professionals involved in a health care team ultimately want the best care and outcomes possible for their patients. Since they will ultimately practice together to achieve this goal, it only makes sense that they learn together.

The concept of teamwork implies engaging both interdependently and collaboratively towards the achievement of a shared, desired outcome. Planning that introduces novice professionals to the interprofessional nature of their work at the pre-service level and then continues to support the continuing professional education and ongoing workplace learning should ultimately strengthen the capacity of sports' health care providers to function as a team. Interprofessional planning at the curricular level, developing courses that cross professions, and structuring rounds in the workplace that highlight the knowledge and skills advanced by all members of the allied professions represented on a team, are ways to build capacity and appropriate translation of knowledge to practice within an existing system.

REFERENCES

Canadian Health Services Research Foundation. (2006). *Teamwork in healthcare: Promoting effective teamwork in healthcare in Canada.* Ottawa: Author.

Canadian Interprofessional Health Collaborative. (2010). *A National Interprofessional Competency Framework.* Vancouver: College of Health Disciplines, University of British Columbia.

Engel, C. (1994). A functional anatomy of teamwork. In A. Leathard (Ed.), *Going interprofessional: Working together for health and welfare.* London: Routledge.

Frank, J.R. (Ed). (2005). *The CanMEDs 2005 physician competency framework: Better standards. Better physicians. Better care.* Ottawa: Royal College of Physicians and Surgeons of Canada.

Frank, J. (2008). Canadian urology programs can be leaders in competency-based education. *Canadian Urology Association Journal, 2*(4), 405.

Frank, J., Jabbour, M., Tugwell, P., Boyd, D., Fréchette, D., Labrosse, J., et al. (1996). *For the societal needs working group. Skills for the new millennium: Report of the societal needs working group.* Ottawa: Royal College of Physicians and Surgeons of Canada.

Government of Ontario. (2005). *Laying the foundation for change. A progress report on Ontario's health human resources initiatives.* Toronto: Author.

Retrieved 10 October 2011 from http://www.health.gov.on.ca/english/
public/pub/ministry_reports/hhr_05/hhr_05.html.

Hall, P., & Weaver, L. (2001). Interdisciplinary education and teamwork:
A long and winding road. *Medical Education, 35,* 867–875.

Orchard, C. (2009). Interprofessional health education and research.
Retrieved 10 September 2009 from http://www.ipe.uwo.ca/about.html.

Sluijs, E.M. (1991). A checklist to assess patient education in physical therapy
practice: Development and reliability. *Physical Therapy, 71*(8), 561–569.

Statistics Canada. (1994). *Adult education and training survey.* Ottawa:
Department of Human Resources and Development, Government of
Canada.

Suter, E., & Deutschlander, S. (2010). Can interprofessional collaboration
provide human resources solutions? A knowledge synthesis. Retrieved
10 October 2011 from http://www.health.heacademy.ac.uk/themes/ipe/
ipe2010/ipcandhhr230310.pdf.

Thomeé, P., Währborg, T., Börjesson, M., Thomeé, R., Eriksson, B., &
Karlsson, J. (2007). Determinants of self-efficacy in the rehabilitation of
patients with anterior cruciate ligament injury. *Journal of Rehabilitative
Medicine, 39,* 486–492.

UNESCO. (1997). The Hamburg Declaration and the agenda for the future.
Hamburg, Germany: UNESCO Institute for Education. Retrieved 10 October
2011 from from http://www.unesco.org/education/uie/confintea/pdf/
con5eng.pdf.

Verma, S., Broers, T., Paerson, M., Schroeder, C., Medves, J., & Morrison, C.
(2009). Core competencies: The next generation comparison of a common
framework for multiple professions. *Journal of Allied Health, 38*(1), 47–54.

World Health Organization. (2009). Increasing access to health workers in
remote and rural areas
through improved retention. Retrieved 10 October 2011 from http://www.
who.int/hrh/migration/background_paper_draft.pdf.

16 Informed Biography as a Focus for Interprofessional Learning: The Case of 'Impaired Driving Causing Death'

KATHRYN HIBBERT, MARK HUNTER,
AND WILLIAM HIBBERT

Interprofessional Education (IPE) is a global movement, driven by factors intent on transforming communities and society in positive ways (Villarreal, 1980; Cribb, 2000; Borrill, West, Shapiro, & Rees, 2000). The Centre for the Advancement of Interprofessional Education (CAIPE) (2002) defines IPE primarily as 'occasions when two or more professions learn from and about each other to improve collaboration and the quality of care' and includes 'learning in academic and work based settings before and after qualification' (n.p.). CAIPE argues that 'no one profession working in isolation has the expertise to respond adequately and effectively to the complexity of many service users "needs"' (n.p.). The goal of IPE is to draw together the experiences of distinct professions to illustrate opportunities for enhancing the overall care and service provided in ways that best prepare professionals within and across disciplines. In separate chapters in this book, Higgs, Trede, and Smith (chapter 14), as well as Gastaldi and Hibbert (chapter 15), also concentrate on interprofessional education.

In this chapter, we present a case of 'Impaired Driving Causing Death' as an illustration of one interprofessional learning context. In the case, we draw together the distinct experiences through a process of first articulating and then analysing the professionally informed biographies of three emergency services personnel involved in a critical incident (a multiple vehicle collision causing death): a paramedic, a police officer, and a nurse.

The power of narrative as a transformative teaching and learning strategy has been well documented (Bruner, 1986, 2002). Narratives, as Randall notes in chapter 11 in this book, offer an authentic rendering of events that engage learners both cognitively and emotionally in ways that invite active meaning making (Clark, 2001). Gathering multiple stories that intersect around a critical incident provides raw material documenting events, offer pre-service learners a process for imagining themselves in a professional role, and in-service learners an opportunity to re-imagine how they collaborate with their emergency services colleagues. Similarly, stories are likely to provoke dialogue and reflection, activities that contribute to improved professional practice (Schön, 1983).

The Case of Impaired Driving Causing Death

Mothers Against Drunk Driving (MADD) Canada (2009) estimates there are between 1,280 and 1,500 impaired crash fatalities in Canada each year (roughly three to four deaths per day), with costs ranging from $2 billion to $12 billion dollars annually. While MADD has focused on educational initiatives aimed at reducing impaired driving, supporting victims, and increasing deterrents, improving the interdisciplinary education of emergency services personnel who respond to these tragedies has received minimal attention. In the following narratives, we aim to provoke new ways to think about practice and planning for interdisciplinary educational possibilities across allied professions. We begin with an overview of the case, and note that all names used are pseudonyms.

'Just the Facts Ma'am'

In March 2001, emergency response units (fire, police, and paramedics) were dispatched to attend a multiple vehicle collision reported by a passing motorist in southwestern Ontario, Canada. The collision between a minivan and a car within a country intersection occurred at approximately 10:30 p.m. Linda and her seven-year-old daughter Melissa were travelling in their family minivan en route to a local school to pick up Melissa's brother from a school dance. At the same time, Brian was travelling alone in his car after a day and night of drinking alcohol at several locations. Brian's vehicle approached a country intersection where it failed to stop at a posted stop sign. Linda's vehicle, travelling on the intersecting roadway not marked with a stop sign, was hit as it entered the intersection. The front of Brian's car collided with the driver's side of the minivan on the intersecting roadway. The force of the collision caused both vehicles to exit the roadway and enter the northwest ditch. When the vehicles came to rest in the ditch, the minivan was on top of the car. Both Linda and Melissa were transported to hospital with critical injuries, and later pronounced deceased. Brian was able to extricate himself from his car and crawl to the roadway where he was discovered by a passing motorist. He was transported to a local hospital and treated for his injuries.

As per protocol, police, firefighters, and paramedics attended the scene. Many of the local volunteer firefighters in attendance knew Linda, Melissa, and their family. The ensuing lengthy investigation by police required, among other things,

- interviews of attending emergency personnel and hospital staff,
- interviews of witnesses (including the passing motorist, but also those who had been drinking with or who had served alcohol to Brian in the preceding hours), and
- writing search warrants and seizing blood samples for alcohol analysis.

As a result of a meticulous investigation, it was determined that Brian's blood alcohol concentration was three times the legal level, and subsequently he was charged with two counts of impaired driving causing death and one count of driving with over the legal limit of alcohol in his blood under the Criminal Code of Canada. Brian subsequently pled guilty and received a four-year prison sentence.

When a collision of this severity occurs, an emergency 911 call unleashes a chain of mandated responses. Routine protocol dictates the dispatch of paramedics, police, and firefighters to the scene, and for hospital personnel to be alerted to probable incoming casualties. Following are three stories that document distinct professional responses to this incident: paramedic, police, and nurse experiences. Articulating and examining the ways in which the three stories unfold and intersect offers a nexus for interprofessional learning overlooked in the chaos of performing individual roles especially in such a highly charged context. Yet, if there are opportunities to improve the ways in which professionals complement and reinforce each other, what better place than in such a demanding context?

The Paramedic Experience

'Unit 4078, code 4, multivictim MVC, intersection of county roads 11 and 9.' En route to the call we were informed that fire was on scene and that there were three patients, all seriously injured.

Suppressing the desire to run up to the scene immediately, I focused my racing mind on the well rehearsed mental checklist. Scene safety first. Where should I park the ambulance so that it will give us protection from traffic and also allow us to leave in a hurry? What hazards exist? Overhead wires? Fuel spills? Traffic? Bystanders? Are the vehicles stable? What forces are involved? What is the speed of the roadway? Remember to note the damage to the vehicles and where they are, as this one is likely going to court. What personal protective equipment do my partner and I need? How many patients are there? Has fire done a sweep of the area to determine if anyone has been ejected or determine if anyone has left the scene? What other resources are required? How can I get access to the patients trapped in the vehicles? Do I send my newbie partner into the vehicle and stay out to coordinate the scene or do I go in and let her handle the rest? Need to remind her that new protocol for termination of resuscitation for patients who are VSA as a result of blunt trauma does not take effect until next month. Leaving the ambulance, I stopped dead in my tracks as I realized that the minivan was the same make, model, and colour as the one my wife drives, but I quickly told myself that she was working evenings and the kids were at my mom's so it couldn't be them. Forcibly repressing that thought, I asked my partner if she would take triage duties.

The fire captain approached my partner and me as we were assembling our gear. I was glad to see that it was Fred, we had worked together often in the past and he was a good guy. Fred said that they discovered three patients; two, a local mother and daughter known to the fire crew are trapped in the van appear critical, and a third, male, found on the roadside 'breathing, with a pulse but unresponsive.' It appeared to Fred that the car blew the stop sign and hit the van. The guy driving the car is alive and 'reeks of booze.' Fighting my initial reaction not to treat the drunk guy, I asked Fred to go with my partner and help her get access to the mother and daughter, and assign a firefighter to me so I could treat the other patient. Before I moved I checked the license plate on the van (thankfully, not mine). A second crew arrives and I direct them to the van to assist with the care of mother and daughter.

I put on my professional face as I approach the drunk who apparently caused this tragedy. Why is it that the innocent ones die and the drunks survive? Despite my personal bias I know I must provide this man with the medical attention he requires. How is my partner doing? Soon I will sit with her and attempt to help her put this together in a manner that will allow her to carry on, both personally and as a medic. The police will want descriptions, observations, thorough notes; I may have to testify. In addition to everything else I need to give thorough attention to what I am observing.

The Police Experience

It was a clear evening in March when I was dispatched to a motor vehicle collision at the intersection of County Road 11 and 9. As I approached the scene, I observed what appeared to be one individual being loaded into an ambulance on a stretcher. As I exited my police vehicle, one of the firefighters ran up to me and told me that there were two female occupants trapped in the minivan, critically injured, and that the driver of the other vehicle had been found on the roadside by a passing motorist. He was the person I had observed in the ambulance. I witnessed firefighters working feverishly around the minivan attempting to extricate its trapped female occupants, who I was told were local and known to the firefighters. Despite the emotionally charged scene, I had to act quickly to secure the area. Were there others who may have been in the crash, ejected, and lying in the ditch? Was there any type of leak from either of the damaged vehicles or possibility of explosion? What evidence is there that will help me determine the cause (and therefore the fault) of this collision? In the absence of poor driving conditions, the presence of drugs and/or alcohol or an underlying medical condition would need to be considered. What do I need to do to establish, document, and control a chain of events and to secure evidence located at the scene of this collision so that it is admissible should this case go to court?

These questions roll around in my head as my experience attending hundreds of serious crashes (and offering evidence during the subsequent legal trials) kicks in. As I help extricate the fatally injured woman and her daughter from the van, I am reminded of my professional responsibility to handle these tasks well. Soon, I will sit with a grief stricken man and his 12-year-old son as they struggle to understand what could have caused the collision that wiped out the other half of their family. They will want answers, and if there was fault on the part of the other driver, they will want justice.

The Nurse Experience

I recall this evening quite well. The ER that night had been steady, but not overly hectic. At about 22:40 hrs we received a call alerting us to a

MVC that had just occurred about 23 km away on a local side road. A passing motorist had found an injured male on the side of the road. He could not tell how many people were in the second vehicle because it was 'in pretty bad shape.'

I let our night doc know we had incoming MVC victims and she asked me to check and see if Lust and Waverly were still in the building to assist. I readied space, meds, and fluids, and moved crash carts into the bays. I was on the phone calling up to the medical floor to let them know we would need additional staff to come down and help us get the patients triaged when a woman from the waiting room started tapping on the window to get my attention. She was concerned that she had been waiting for nearly an hour to see a doctor. I bluntly told her that she'll be waiting a lot longer than that, then immediately regretted my tone. I alerted X-ray and started the requisite documentation. I found myself stealing glances at the clock and the door while trying to maintain the flow of patient care already in progress. Although we are well-trained to think quickly and perform our tasks professionally, I can't avoid the creeping 'what ifs' that linger in the corners of my mind. What if I know the victims? Where is my husband and our son right now? My thoughts are interrupted by a patient in the second bay who needs a bed pan, but before I get to her, I have to go over her orders with the doc.

At that moment the doors swing open and we move into high gear. The first two to arrive are a mother and daughter. The paramedics are speaking quickly: Female. 39, VSA. Extricated from her vehicle with visible head and chest trauma. Attempts to resuscitate en route unsuccessful. We help them move the patient into the bay bed and check for a pulse, any breath sounds. One of the docs calls the death and immediately joins her colleague in the next bay who has taken over CPR on the second female victim, aged seven, extricated from the same vehicle. When resuscitation efforts fail, she too is pronounced dead.

As we are processing the gravity of the situation a third victim is brought in. Male, 46, awake but disoriented. My heart sinks as the smell of alcohol is immediately detected. I suppress the overwhelming feeling that threatens to overtake my need to remain professional. The police officer at the door signals a likely impaired. I know that they have to notify the victims' families, and I register that they will also need a statement from me about the third victim. I smelled alcohol. They will want a blood sample that has to be collected, labelled, and stored according to their protocol in the likely event that there is a court case. My mind quickly snaps back to the care and treatment of the patient. His vital signs are good. His injuries appear minor. The docs have ordered a cleaning and dressing of a few minor abrasions. I find myself fighting to stay professional. The husband and father of the female victims have just arrived. The woman from the waiting room taps on the window again ... 'I've been waiting an awfully long time,' she says.

The Intersection of Knowledge/Skills

Looking across the three informed biographies prompted several questions: How have we, as professionals who interact with emergency services colleagues regularly over many years, maintained such a level of ignorance about the intricacies of each others' roles? What assumptions are implicit in our interactions? How might role clarification and interprofessional learning opportunities reduce duplication and improve our respective services? Where do opportunities for what we believe to be rich learning fit into the lives of busy professionals?

Jarvis (2003) has documented the importance of experiential learning in contexts in which we are required to 'think on our feet.' What distinguishes the emergency services personnel in this case is that they all practise in contexts which are frequently chaotic, complex, and emotionally charged. In addition, their sites of practise are shifting; from the scene, to the ambulance, to various areas of a hospital, to a courtroom. Decisions made 'in the moment' are governed by particular protocols in place for each profession, but could be later scrutinized or questioned. They are also informed by the individual contexts, prior experiences, and assumptions that each professional brings to the encounter.

In the study of paramedics working in such highly charged, non-fixed environments, Campeau (2008) posits an interesting 'space control theory,' suggesting that emergency personnel learn to 'adapt themselves and the environment around the patient ... [and] achieve this adaptation by controlling the activities that take place in the space immediately around the patient' (pp. 288–289). Citing Milligan (1998), Campeau further argues that emergencies represent sites of 'interactional potential' creating a "multicrisis' [where] managing these scenes requires what can be characterized as interactionist detective work' (p. 291). We draw on this notion of interactionist detective work to uncover the interactional potential for multidisciplinary, professionally informed biographies to serve interprofessional education needs.

Interactionist Detective Work

A close look at the three narratives reveals that an identified protocol for professional practice is in place for each of the emergency services professions. By positioning the narratives alongside each other and considering their governing protocols (see Table 16.1), it becomes clear that they present a nexus for collaboration and learning that, unexamined,

Table 16.1. An Overview of Responsibilities Enacted in a Single Case

Police responsibilities	Paramedic responsibilities	Nurse responsibilities
Secure and take control of collision scene	Secure and take control of shifting scene	Control shifting scene in hospital
Assess scene (injuries, potential for hazards, explosions, etc.)	Assess scene (injuries, potential for hazards, explosions etc.)	Assess hospital scene and prepare to receive patients
Decisions about resources needed	Decisions about resources needed	Decisions about resources needed
Set priorities for flow of tasks and gather information from paramedics, fire, witnesses	Set priorities and gather information from police, fire, witnesses	Set priorities and gather information from paramedics, police, family in attendance
Ensuring flow of response (emergency vehicles, communication with family, victims, etc.)	Communicate with patients and hospital staff, ensure safe and efficient transport and transfer	Communicate with hospital staff, family, and ensure flow of treatment
Maintain security of the scene and assist with extrication of victims / collect scene evidence	Assess and treat patients / coordinate extrication with fire	Perform diagnostic tests and treatment or confirm and pronounce death
Track where victims are taken, follow up to continue to gather and preserve evidence	Determine transport priority, and ascertain most appropriate receiving facility	
Conduct appropriate follow-up investigation.	Review procedures	
Documentation	Documentation	Documentation

may result in a collision of misconceptions, power struggles, and missed opportunities to serve patients better. As such, narratives that wrap a critical incident like this offer rich sites for both professional and inter-professional learning in a variety of contexts: universities, colleges, on the job training, staff meetings, or individual professional reading.

Returning to our case example, we note that each professional has been trained to establish control of the scene and to create a sense of organization within the chaos. For example, the objectives for controlling the scene overlap for the police and paramedics where safety issues are concerned, as they assess for hazards, determine the number of victims involved, and attempt to minimize the risks to victims and responders. Although a collaborative and collegial approach to the scene is preferred, the reality of distinct disciplines attempting to achieve similar and overlapping objectives with minimal understanding of each other's capability and responsibility within the context of an emotionally charged environment may result in conflict and reduced effectiveness. Such overlapping practices, and protocol presents an ideal place to begin interprofessional education and training where a common set of knowledge skills and practices could align and improve the seamless interaction between allied professionals. At the same time, learning about the focus, protocols, and communication of each other where their activities do not align, can serve to promote understanding and insight into ways they may be able to further improve the interactions.

The specifics of their distinct mandates vary somewhat, but are embedded in each role. The scene in this type of critical incident is a shifting one. For police, the scene includes the physical space (in this case the intersecting roadways and damaged vehicles) where evidence is preserved, photographed, measured, and collected. As those involved in the incident are moved from the scene, police must follow that movement to continue their investigation. For paramedics, the scene is the patient and the area directly surrounding the patient. Their interest in controlling the physical space is entirely related to its impact on the health and well-being of the patient. They relinquish all care and concern for the physical space once all injured are in transport. Upon arrival at the hospital, they relinquish control a second time. Control transfers to the triage nurse who has been preparing the hospital site to receive incoming patients. Like her professional colleagues in the field, she must determine what resources are needed, assess the site for potential explosions (the emotionally charged, sometimes illegal substance variety), and manage the care efficiently and effectively in the midst of what is very often a chaotic setting. The scene continues to shift, as injured are often moved to various locations within the hospital setting for diagnosis and treatment. In situations where impaired driving is suspected, police must maintain control of the shifting scene as they gather evidence; in this case, the legal search and seizure of blood samples.

To What End?

As previously noted, a global movement towards interprofessional education in health care continues to gain momentum as a means of coping with the acknowledged complexities and challenges. However despite complex, regular interactions between emergency services personnel and overlapping responsibilities as illustrated in the above case, minimal progress has been made to implement interprofessional education within emergency services. How might interprofessional socialization and education serve the overall goal of improving services? For example, if Emergency Services personnel were to come together around an authentic case study like this impaired case, what difference would it make to the ways in which paramedics and nurses documented their notes after glimpsing the role their information plays in the successful prosecution of a case? Patient confidentiality precludes paramedics and nurses verbally sharing with police information that may be vital to their investigation. However, police can obtain documentation from paramedics and nursing staff under the authority of a search warrant that then allows the information to be considered for legal proceedings. How might understanding the process more fully inform the time and effort put into the meticulous documentation of notes from a scene by busy professionals?

The practice of adult education has been long seen as a 'place of social transformation' (Schroeder, 1999, p. xiii). Although often separated into formal and informal contexts, learning occurs in both places. The challenge with informal and 'on the job' contexts is that learning can be sporadic and undisciplined (p. 76) thereby failing to avail itself of practices that may ensure transformational outcomes from the learning. Given the competing demands of the working day, this is understandable if unsatisfactory. As Barr, Koppel, Reeves, Hammick, and Freeth (2005) have noted, the rising public expectations, dwindling resources, and increased workplace complexities can lead to increased occupational stress (p. 10). In order to bring together professionals who have imperfect understandings of their interdependent relationships with one another in ways that better serve the public and the participating professionals, we posed the following questions:

- What principles might be developed for interprofessional learning in a context like this?
- What form and function might conversations across the professions take?
- What issues around professional identity arise as the professions intersect?
- How might existing 'silo' curricula be modified to embrace interprofessional education?
- What does it mean to move interprofessional knowledge about education into a broader professional community?
- What are the challenges involved in coordinating the learning of multiple emergency services personnel? What are the opportunities?
- In what way do the current cultures support or inhibit interprofessional learning?
- How do we create champions within each organization?
- How might we each press for more interdisciplinary links in our work as adult educators?
- How do we coordinate continuing education credits (different requirements/expectations across organizations)?
- What role might e-learning play in the response and why?

Ethically Responsible Action

As we considered the questions that were raised in our examination of our stories, we draw on principles of adult education that focus on core competency development. Core competencies such as communication, teamwork, self-direction, and reflection may offer flexible ways that communities of professionals may elect to engage in as part of their pre-service and continuing in-service education. In the context of our case study, we consider these core competencies and suggest possibilities for interprofessional teaching and learning.

In *After Virtue*, philosopher Alasdair McIntyre (1984) claims, 'I can only answer the question, "What am I to do?" if I can answer the prior question, "Of what story or stories do I find myself a part?"' (p. 216). A useful exercise for educators and students at all levels would be to consider what stories they are a part of as a means of situating their practice within the broader context of authentic experience. Certainly it is useful to develop discipline-specific knowledge and skills; however, distinct knowledge and skills are not applied in an isolated context. Professionals, as illustrated in the case example here, often practice in community not in isolation.

A reasonable adaptation to any course would be an exercise that situates their training within an interdisciplinary context that requires an understanding of how the parts operate as a whole. This could be achieved through a number of means:

- Curriculum mapping with a view to looking for potential interprofessional teaching opportunities:
  - For example, documentation. How might documentation conducted by related services better align or be developed to ensure that it meets the needs of all involved?
- Faculty Development:
  - In what ways might faculty development sessions include a 'role play' of stories like the one offered in this case as a means of stimulating dialogue about how constituent professions might better work together?
- Action Learning:
  - How might cases such as this one be used to create 'observational guides' for pre-service students during a practicum, or in-service professionals during a review or debriefing process?
- Teamwork:
  - How might interdisciplinary groups work on projects that allow them to investigate and analyse issues related to cases like this? How might this reposition learners as problem solvers and serve to disrupt assumptions?
- Continuing Professional Education:
  - How might allied professionals work together to create continuing learning opportunities that meet their shared needs? For example, accessing a collaborative website that offers cases like this with examples of how each of the emergency services professions viewed their 'care and control' roles may stimulate reflection on action (Schön, 1983) in ways that lead to a deeper understanding of how they might function better together, and demonstrate respect for the skill set, needs, and mandate each brings to the incident.

Conclusion

This chapter has explored interprofessional collaborative teaching and learning opportunities revealed in the nexus of the informed biographies of three distinct emergency services professions: paramedicine, policing, and nursing. The case identified a common set of core competencies across these professions as well as locations in which responsibilities intersect. Opportunities for interdisciplinary training are presented where interprofessional education can be advanced for emergency service professionals. Examples within the training context include: curriculum mapping, faculty development, action learning, teamwork, and continuing professional education. One of the most productive outcomes, from the perspective of the authors, has been the dialogue that surrounded a single critical incident. Taking the time to share and then interrogate our multiple perspectives has been highly instructive to deepening our individual and collective understandings of the important roles that we each play as we work in service of the public.

REFERENCES

Barr, H., Koppel, I., Reeves, S., Hammick, M., & Freeth, D. (2005). *Effective interprofessional education: Argument, assumption, and evidence.* Oxford: Blackwell Publishing.

Borrill, C.,West, M., Shapiro, D., & Rees, A. (2000). Team working and effectiveness in healthcare. *British Journal of Health Care Management, 6*(8), 364–371.

Bruner, J. (1986). *Actual minds, possible worlds.* Cambridge, MA: Harvard University Press.

Bruner, J. (2002). *Making stories.* New York: Farrar, Strauss, and Giroux.

CAIPE. (2002). Centre for the Advancement of Interprofessional Education. Retrieved 10 October 2011 from http://www.caipe.org.uk/.

Campeau, A.G. (2008). The space control theory of paramedic scene management. *Symbolic Interaction, 31* (3), 285-302.

Clark, M.C. (2001). Off the beaten path: Some creative approaches to adult learning. In S.B. Merriam (Ed.), *The new update on adult learning theory. New directions in adult and continuing education, 89.* San Francisco: Jossey-Bass.

Cribb, A. (2000). The diffusion of the health agenda and the fundamental need for partnership in medical education. *Medical Education, 34,* 916–920.

Jarvis, P. (2003). Adult education and lifelong learning: Theory and practice, 93. Retrieved 10 October 2011 from http://www.myilibrary.com/Browse/open.asp?ID=7796&loc=101.

MADD Canada. (2009). Estimating the presence of alcohol and drug impairment in traffic crashes and their costs to Canadians. MADD Canada Research Library. Retrieved 10 October 2011 from http://www.madd.ca/english/research/estimating_presence.pdf.

McIntyre, A. (1984). *After virtue.* Notre Dame, IN: Notre Dame University Press.

Schön, D. (1983). *The reflective practitioner: How professionals think in action.* London: Temple Smith.

Schroeder, S. (1999). *The metaphysics of cooperation: A case study of F.D. Maurice.* Amsterdam: Rodopi.

Villarreal, R. (1980). Universidad Autónoma Metropolitana, Xochimilco, Mexico: An interdisciplinary innovation in medical education. *Public Health Papers, 2*(1), 71–80.

PART IV

Conclusion

17 Closing Reflections

LEONA M. ENGLISH

This book has brought together a number of professionals in the areas of health and adult learning to share elements of their practice and to contribute to a growing knowledge basis on the intersection of these seemingly disparate areas. Collectively, the writers – from fields as varied as adult education, nursing, medicine, sports therapy, and occupational therapy – have contributed to an emergent field of practice that was called adult health learning in chapter 1, a field that has the potential to transform how we work and how we interact when it comes to issues of health.

One of the key themes arising from this book is an affirmation that much significant learning occurs at the community level, by ordinary citizens both on their own and in conjunction with health and other workers in the community. Adult learning happens in the community when adults come together to make decisions about issues that affect their health, and when they take responsibility for acting on their innate knowledge of matters that affect them. Part I of the book made this case by pointing first to the critical issues that determine health – geography, culture, employment, gender, and so on – and to how these dimensions cannot be isolated from the need to access adequate health and medical services. Part II then worked to provide cases and to address issues in the context of community. What comes through in these community-based cases is that lifelong learning is a necessity for a healthy community and that communities never stop growing and learning – they need to work collectively to build their knowledge base and to broaden their scope to areas well beyond medical systems. The various authors emphasize that adult learning principles and theories have much to offer in creating linkages to the community, organizing for analysis and action, and

in affecting healthy public policy around health. Adult educators bring
their skill and knowledge base acquired from time spent mapping the
assets of communities and working with participants to build a collective
future.

It is also true, however, that significant learning happens in higher education and in formal clinical settings. The authors in Part III addressed
the ongoing education of professionals in such settings. They were concerned with how these professionals are educated as well as with the content of their education and field of practice. Whether one is teaching
nurses or gerontologists, many of the crucial issues are similar: culture,
gender, skills, and context. The overarching theme in this section is that
the exclusivist and medical model has served us in a limited way in our
teaching situations. In its focus on the transmission of knowledge, it has
been shown to have limited long-term durability. The authors here have
shown that if the educational encounter involves learners as participants
it will more likely be effective. And, if it involves a strong critically reflective practice component and an approach that is interdisciplinary it is
more likely to be effective long term. The illustrative cases and exercises
in these chapters encourage collaboration, dialogue, and person-centred
earning, all cornerstones of the adult education field.

Emerging in the chapters in Part III is a transformational view of health
learning which the authors have found useful and have worked hard
to develop in their own areas of practice in education and continuing
professional education contexts. They see learning about health as part
of a continuum of knowledge that engages participants, communities,
and experts working together to transform health and make system-wide
change that ultimately addresses health needs that have been identified
in participatory ways.

In presenting a variety of authors from a number of different professions and countries, this book has shown the spectrum of persons
interested in a renewed vision of health that moves beyond a liberal
teaching model and which embraces democratic and participatory ways
of knowing. Indeed, the authors have endeavoured to challenge liberal
and transmission models of teaching and to bring them into conversation with critical ideas such as the community as knowers; researchers
as community partners; and professionals as interprofessional team
workers. In sharing examples from their own practice the authors have
challenged tired models of expert knowledge and replaced them with
models that are analytical and challenging, and which contribute to long-
term change and community empowerment. Theirs is a lifelong learning

approach that reaches from assessing the environmental impact of living in contaminated areas to being actively involved in food production in a local area. The authors are on the vanguard of change in thinking about a transformational view of adult health learning, one that points to the development of a learning culture in health which honours the full spectrum of learning from informal to formal and nonformal.

Yet, for all that has been proposed, there remain some burning questions about how to broaden the audience of health and learning, to policy-makers and government leaders, to deans of education, and to professional associations, all of whom affect teaching and learning for health. This issue of policy is an important one, yet it seems to quite illusory in this area, perhaps because of the enormous energy and effort exerted on behalf of medical systems and expert knowledge. Until decision-makers and policy experts make the shift to a comprehensive view of healthy communities, which necessitates honouring people as knowers and indigenous knowledge as valid, many of these ideas and practices will be ineffective. When this link is made, health and learning will become more of a reality.

A related question remains about the willingness of professions to acknowledge that interdisciplinary work and learning from areas such as education can be of benefit to them and the patients in their care. While a great deal of effort is already ongoing to work in interprofessional teams and to do collective continuing education, as the authors in this book evidence, there is still resistance to moving to a more participatory framework. Transitions are difficult, and yet they seem to be essential if a transformational model of health and learning are deemed possible.

Yet, with the 29 contributors of this book a modest effort has been made to strengthen the links between health and learning, community and experts, official and indigenous knowledge. Although the project is long term, it is worth the effort.

Glossary

Aboriginal is a term applied to status and non-status Indians, Inuvialuit, Inuit, and Métis. 'Aboriginal' is the term used in the Canadian Constitution.

African indigenous knowledge is locally based knowledge that is generated through a systematic process of observing the local environments, experimenting with solutions, and the re-adopting of previously identified solutions to changing environmental factors.

Autobiographical learning is a variation on 'learning from experience.' Autobiographical learning involves learning about ourselves and from ourselves through reflection on the memories and stories in terms of which we have constructed our identity across the years. Autobiographical learning is something we may be especially capable of and open to in later life.

Biographical aging is an aspect of aging not normally considered in mainstream gerontology. Biographical aging – in contrast to biological aging – concerns how we age and change, subjectively or psychologically, with respect to how we experience ourselves over time.

Communities of practice are communities or groups in a particular discipline or setting working together, setting norms and expectations of practice, and participating in the framing of each community. A key feature of these communities is that learning is embedded in practice rather than being a separate or optional activity (Higgs, Ajjawi, & Smith, 2009).

Community development is the process of developing active and sustainable communities that are based on social justice and mutual respect. Whether community development happens internationally or domestically, it involves influencing power structures to remove the barriers that prevent people from participating in issues that affect their lives. Education and empowerment are core concepts in community development (Federation for Community Development Learning, 2007).

Community Health Impact Assessment (CHIA) is a facilitated process that engages a community in developing a unique assessment tool, and empowers that community to initiate its own impact assessment with that tool regarding issues such as development that affect their health. Both the assessment tool and the assessment process reflect the community's values, beliefs, and visions of what a healthy community should look like (NCCHPP, 2009).

Community-engaged research is a process of inclusive and authentic participation between academics and community members to address issues affecting mutual well-being. Community engaged research is enacted through partnerships, collaborative arrangements, and coalitions that help mobilize resources and influence systems, and serve as catalysts for changing policies, programs, and practices (Jones & Wells, 2007; Minkler & Wallerstein, 2008).

Curriculum mapping is a process that reviews curricula to identify key elements such as knowledge, skills, competencies, and main issues. It is used both vertically by individual teachers (e.g., to inform planning, to document and compare differences between the planned curriculum and the enacted curriculum), and horizontally across organizations to reduce duplication and to ensure key competencies are addressed in a multifaceted program.

First Nations are the indigenous nations who existed in North America before the arrival of the European explorers. This term can refer to a single band, or sometimes, to a group of bands affiliated with a tribal council or cultural group. Although some apply the term First Nations to all aboriginal people of Canada (Indians, Inuit, Inuvialuit, and Métis) many aboriginal people prefer to be recognized for the specific band or First Nation to which they belong. Others prefer to be identified according to tribal or cultural grouping.

Harm reduction is an approach to health promotion that emphasizes the reduction of harmful consequences associated with certain behaviours, when the cessation of such behaviours is not tenable in the short term. Sexual behaviours (condom use) and substance use (needle exchange) are both examples of a harm reduction approach. Harm reduction policies, programs, and practices subscribe to a non-judgmental approach that respects the dignity of individuals to make their own choices about their use. Harm reduction strategies include education (e.g., learning about the health consequences associated with drug use), and the development of community-based facilities (e.g., needle-exchange sites).

Health is defined by the World Health Organization as: 'A state of complete physical, social and mental well-being, and not merely the absence of disease or infirmity' (WHO, 1986, p. 1). The WHO sees health as a resource for everyday life, not the objective of living. Health is a positive concept emphasizing social and personal resources, as well as physical capacities (WHO, 1998).

Health education comprises consciously constructed opportunities for learning involving some form of communication designed to improve health literacy, including improving knowledge and developing life skills which are conducive to individual and community health (WHO, 1998).

Health Impact Assessment (HIA) is a combination of procedures, methods, and tools that systematically judges the potential and sometimes unintended effects of a policy, plan, program, or project on the health of a population and the distribution of those effects within the population. HIA identifies appropriate actions to manage those effects (IAIA, 2006).

Health promotion represents the process of enabling people to increase control over, and to improve, their health. It is a comprehensive social and political process that not only embraces actions directed at strengthening the skills and capabilities of individuals, but is also action directed towards changing social, environmental, and economic conditions so as to alleviate their impact on public and individual health. Participation is essential to sustain health promotion action (WHO, 1998).

Healthy public policy is policy that increases the health and well-being of those individuals whom it affects (Kemm, 2001). It is public policy that potentially enhances a population's health by having a positive impact on the social, economic, and environmental determinants of health. This approach is based on the understanding that health is influenced by many factors, such as education, social support, income, and the physical environment. Public policies regarding issues such as transportation and housing are tools to influence these determinants of health. (NCCHPP, 2008).

Indigenous people is a term used by the United Nations to refer to aboriginal peoples in any area of the world.

Indigenousness, within an African context, refers to the traditional norms, social values, and mental constructs that guide, organize, and regulate African ways of living in making sense to the world.

Interprofessional education refers to the process whereby members from two or more professions, or students preparing to enter practice in a variety of professions, learn together to improve their practice of patient care (CAIPE, 2007).

Narrative care is a concept developed within the framework of a narrative gerontology. Narrative care – expressible in various ways, through various strategies – entails a fundamental respect for the storied complexity of those for whom we care, whatever their situation and whatever the context in which we work (e.g., acute care, palliative care, long-term care).

Narrative gerontology is an emerging sub-field within gerontology that reflects the impact of the narrative turn throughout the social sciences. Narrative gerontology is rooted in the assumption that human beings are meaning-making beings and that our main means of making it is through telling, interpreting, and exchanging stories. Key themes in narrative gerontology are the storied complexity of identity, memory, and experience in later life – including the experience of aging itself.

Population health refers to the health of a population as measured by health status indicators and as influenced by social, economic, and physical environments; personal health practices; individual capacity and coping skills; human biology; early childhood development; and health services. Population health proponents focus on the variety and interconnections of factors that influence the health, identify variations in their patterns of occurrence, and implement policies and actions based on this knowledge. (The Federal, Provincial, Territorial Advisory Committee on Population Health, 1994).

Public health is a collective and societal effort to sustain and promote the people's health. Public health builds on expert and community knowledge, and involves programs, services, and institutions to help in preventing disease and promoting health.

Stages of change, or the *Transtheoretical Model,* was developed by James Prochaska and Carlo DiCelemente. This model of health behaviour change highlights the role of individual readiness, indicating that change is an internal process (as opposed to one that can be externally imposed). Different issues and tasks are related to each of six stages – precontemplation, contemplation, preparation, action, maintenance, and termination – through which individuals progress in a spiraling fashion with relapse identified as a normal and expected part of the process. The model has been applied to a range of health behaviours, including substance use, eating disorders, and weight loss.

REFERENCES

CAIPE (Centre for the Advancement of Interprofessional Education). (2007). Definition of interprofessional education. Retrieved 20 July 2007 from www. caipe.org.uk.

Federal/Provincial/Territorial Advisory Committee on Population Health. (1994). *Strategies for population health: Investing in the health of Canadians.* Ottawa: Health and Welfare Canada. Retrieved 17 May 2010 from http:// www.phac-aspc.gc.ca/ph-sp/pdf/strateg-eng.pdf.

Federation for Community Development Learning. (2007). A definition of community development. Retrieved 15 September 2009 from http://www. fcdl.org.uk/about/definition.htm.

Higgs, J., Ajjawi, R., & Smith, M. (2009). Working and learning in communities of practice. In J. Higgs, M. Smith, G. Webb, M. Skinner, & A. Croker (Eds.), *Contexts of physiotherapy practice* (pp. 117–127). Melbourne: Elsevier Australia.

IAIA (International Association of Impact Assessment). (2006). *Health impact assessment: International best practice principles.* Special publication series no. 5. Retrieved 10 October 2011 from http://www.iaia.org/publicdocuments/ special-publications/SP5.pdf.

Jones L., & Wells K. (2007). Strategies for academic and clinician engagement in community-participatory partnered research. *JAMA, 297,* 407–410.

Kemm, J. (2001). Health impact assessment: A tool for healthy public policy. *Health Promotion International, 16*(1), 79–85.

Minkler, M., & Wallerstein, N. (Eds.). (2008). *Community-based participatory research for health: From process to outcomes* (2d ed.). San Francisco: Jossey-Bass.

NCCHPP (National Collaborating Centre for Healthy Public Policy). (2008). Healthy public policy: How do public policies affect health? What does research tell us? Retrieved 1 October 2010 from http://www.ccnpps.ca/548/ Healthy+Public+Policy.htm.

NCCHPP. (National Collaborating Centre on Healthy Public Policy). (2009). Influencing healthy public policy with community Health Impact Assessment. Retrieved 10 October 2011 from http://www.ccnpps.ca/docs/PATH_ Rapport_EN.pdf.

World Health Organization (WHO). (1986). Ottawa charter for health promotion. Retrieved 2 March 2009 from http://www.who.int/hpr/archive/docs/ottawa.html.

World Health Organization (WHO). (1998). Health promotion glossary. Retrieved 10 October from http://www.who.int/hpr/NPH/docs/hp_glossary_en.pdf.

Contributors

Marlene Atleo, ʔehʔeh naa tuu kwiss, Nuu-chah-nulth, Ahousaht First Nation, is an associate professor at the University of Manitoba, Winnipeg, where she coordinates the adult and post-secondary program and writes in the areas of aboriginal health, institutional development, and post-secondary education.

Stephen Brookfield is distinguished university professor at the University of St. Thomas in Minneapolis-St. Paul, MN. He is a four-time winner of the Cyril O. Houle World Award for Literature in Adult Education and has written or co-edited 13 books on adult learning, critical thinking, teaching, discussion methods, and critical theory.

Colleen Cameron is a senior program teaching staff member at the Coady International Institute, and a clinical associate in the School of Nursing at St. Francis Xavier University, Antigonish, NS. She has been involved in research and training of NGO staff and volunteers in the PATH process in India, Ghana, and Sierra Leone, as well as in Canada.

Marie-Ève Caty is a speech-language pathologist and PhD student in health professional education at the University of Western Ontario, London. Her strong interest in continuing professional development and research has led her to become interested in researching reflective practice.

Bagele Chilisa is an associate professor at the University of Botswana, Gaborone, where she teaches research and evaluation courses. She researches HIV prevention education and methodologies that are inclusive of African indigenous ways of knowing, perceiving reality, and value systems. She is co-author of *Research Methods for Adult Educators in Africa*.

Donna M. Chovanec is an associate professor of adult education in educational policy studies at the University of Alberta, Edmonton. She has experience as a social worker, adult educator, and researcher in health and social service settings. She is especially interested in the learning experiences of marginalized adults. She is the author of *Between Hope and Despair: Women Learning Politics*.

Maureen Coady is assistant professor in the Adult Education Department, Saint Francis Xavier University, Antigonish, NS. Her research focuses on the links between health and learning, and the role of adult education in enabling people to take action related to their health. She is currently examining learning experienced by health professionals and adult learners when health promotion/education programs are delivered in community settings.

John P. Egan is senior manager, curriculum counselling, in the Centre for Teaching, Learning and Technology at the University of British Columbia, Vancouver. His work has been published in *The Journal of Interprofessional Care*, the *International Dictionary of Adult Education*, and the *Handbook of Adult and Continuing Education*. John holds a PhD in educational studies (adult education) from the University of British Columbia.

Leona M. English is professor in the Department of Adult Education at St. Francis Xavier University. Her writing and research are mainly in the areas of spirituality, poststructuralism, and gender and learning. She edited the *International Encyclopedia of Adult Education*.

Brian Gastaldi is a registered physiotherapist with 27 years of experience. He has served on the Canadian Medical Therapy Team in five Olympics and holds a diploma in sport physical therapy. He is former director of physiotherapy at the Fowler-Kennedy Sport Medicine Clinic, University of Western Ontario, London. He is currently in private practice.

Kathryn Hibbert is an assistant professor at the Faculty of Education and the Schulich School of Medicine and Dentistry at the University of Western Ontario. She has served as founding director of the Centre for

Education in Medical Imaging, director of continuing teacher education, and is a core member of INPiRE, an interdisciplinary network for scholarship in professions research in education.

William Hibbert, BA, BEd, is a provincial police sergeant serving Western Region, ON. As lead reconstructionist, he investigated 359 serious/fatal motor vehicle collisions and serves as an expert in the field at all court levels. He has been an author/instructor of regional collision training programs, community college traffic programs, and police recruits at the Ontario Police College. He is currently completing graduate studies in adult education.

Joy Higgs, AM, BSc, MHPEd, PhD, is strategic research professor in professional practice, and director at the Education for Practice Institute at Charles Sturt University, Sydney, Australia. Joy has worked in higher education for more than 26 years and received a Member of the Order of Australia award for her contributions to this field. She has produced over 400 publications, including over 20 books.

Mark Hunter, AEMCA, RN, BScN, is a registered nurse and paramedic educator at Fanshawe College in London, ON. He has served as an expert witness for paramedic education and led the curriculum development for paramedicpPrograms in Ontario. He serves on the Emergency Health Services Paramedic Advisory Committee and has received national awards for teaching excellence. Mark is completing graduate studies in education.

Karen Jenkins has worked at the Middlesex-London Health Unit in Ontario for 17 years. Her current position involves coordinating student placements. Karen is currently completing her master's in health and rehabilitative sciences with an interest in preceptor education and reflective practice.

Brettany Johnson is a doctoral student in educational policy studies at the University of Alberta, Edmonton, and a project manager at the Centre for Health Evidence. She has experience working in a broad range of health education contexts. Her research interests include workplace learning, practitioner research, and knowledge translation. Recent projects include *Evidence Access: Shaping Knowledge Transfer in Rural Alberta*.

Elizabeth Anne Kinsella is an associate professor in health sciences and women's studies at the University of Western Ontario, London. She is co-director of the Interdisciplinary Network for Scholarship in Professions' Research in Education and a researcher with The Centre for Education Research and Innovation, at Western. Her scholarship is located in the area of reflection and health professional education.

Jane Moseley is an assistant professor, School of Nursing, St. Francis Xavier University, Antigonish, NS. With 25 years' practice in community, Jane currently teaches population-focused community health nursing. Her research areas are improving teaching-learning strategies, enhancing public health nursing through population health partnerships, and developing equity opportunities for aboriginal and black Nova Scotia students in undergraduate nursing education.

Stella Ng is an audiologist and CIHR-STIHR fellow in health care, technology, and place at the University of Toronto. Her practice experiences as an educational audiologist led her to research interest in student clinicians' use of reflection in their development as professional practitioners.

Peggy Gabo Ntseane is an associate professor in adult education at the University of Botswana, Gaborone. She holds a BSc and MA in sociology, as well as a graduate certificate in gender studies and a PhD in adult education. Her HIV/AIDS research experience includes prevention education, culture, transformational learning, and behavioural change.

Dan Pratt is professor of adult and higher education, Department of Educational Studies, and senior scholar in health professions education in the Faculty of Medicine, University of British Columbia, Vancouver. In 1999 his book, *Five Perspectives on Teaching in Adult and Higher Education*, won the Cyril O. Houle Award for Literature in Adult Education. In 2008 he received Canada's most prestigious university teaching award: the 3M National Teaching Fellowship.

William Randall is professor of gerontology at St. Thomas University in Fredericton, NB. He has published extensively on narrative gerontology and related themes in such periodicals as *Narrative Inquiry, Theory and Psychology,* the *McGill Journal of Education,* and the *Canadian Journal on Aging.* His most recent book, with Elizabeth McKim, is *Reading Our Lives: The Poetics of Growing Old* (Oxford, 2008).

Barbara Ronson is an independent educator and consultant currently working with the Aboriginal Studies program at the University of Toronto and with the Ontario Healthy Schools Coalition.

Irving Rootman, PhD, is a former professor and Michael Smith Foundation for Health Research distinguished scholar at the University of Victoria, BC. He has done research in health promotion for more than 30 years and has focused mainly on literacy and health for the past 10 years.

Leslie Sadownik is an obstetrician/gynecologist with a master's degree in adult education. She is director of the UBC Faculty Development Program and an assistant professor in the Department of Ob/Gyn. She has received numerous teaching awards, including UBC Clinical Faculty Excellence in Teaching Award, the Association of Canadian Medical Colleges Young Educator Award, and the Association of Professors of Obstetrics and Gynecology Excellence in Teaching Award.

Sandra Jarvis Selinger is an assistant professor in the Department of Surgery and associate director in the eHealth Strategy Office, University of British Columbia, Vancouver. She is a PhD-trained educational specialist and researcher in the area of human learning, development, and instruction at the UBC Faculty of Education. Her work focuses on innovation and knowledge translation in medical education. In 2008 she received a Michael Smith Foundation for Health Research Career Investigator Award.

Megan Smith, BAppSc (physio); MAppSc (cardiopulmary physio), PhD, is a senior lecturer at Charles Sturt University, Sydney, Australia. She leads the physiotherapy program and has been involved in the program at CSU since 1999. She is currently the sub-dean for professional placements for the Faculty of Science. Her teaching and research interests are cardiorespiratory physiotherapy practice, clinical education, and clinical reasoning.

Franziska Trede, DipPhty, MHPEd, PhD, is senior lecturer in the Education for Practice Institute at Charles Sturt University, Sydney, Australia. She has worked in higher education for more than 13 years with a focus on intercultural communication, health beliefs, and behaviour change, clinical education, health promotion, and learning and teaching. Her research interest is in the educational dimension of health care practice.

Linda Ziegahn, PhD, co-leads the Community Engagement Program for the Clinical and Translational Science Center at the University of California, Davis, where she works to forge partnerships between health researchers and community members. Her research interests focus on the role of learning in community-engaged health research and on critical reflection around cultural learning.